HEALING STORIES

TO INSPIRE, TEACH & HEAL

True Stories About
Giving, Receiving, Teaching & Learning
Energy-Based Care

Mary Jo Bulbrook

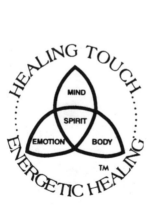

Healing Touch Partnerships, Inc.
Carrboro, North Carolina

Healing Stories: To Inspire, Teach and Heal

Published by
North Carolina Center for Healing Touch
Publishing Division
Healing Touch Partnerships, Inc.
413 Waterside Drive
Carrboro, NC 27510-1290
Phone: (919) 942-5214
Fax: (919) 968-0994
e-mail: maryjo@mindspring.com
www.mindspring.com/~maryjo

© 2000 by Mary Jo Bulbrook

Edited by Dan Trollinger

ISBN:1-889293-09-1

Dr. Mary Jo Bulbrook (RN, CHTP, CHTI) is the Founder and Director of Healing Touch Partnerships, Inc., a worldwide organization dedicated to Connecting through the Light. Detailed information about this organization is listed in the Appendix.

Cost: $20

Printed in USA

TABLE OF CONTENTS

CONNECTING WITH HEART AND HANDS

Chapter 1   Clinical Vignettes

Chapter 2   Family Healing Stories

Chapter 2   Family Healing Stories (Continued)

Chapter 3   Case Studies

Chapter 4   Teaching & Learning Energy-Based Therapy

CONNECTING WITH ANIMALS AND LAND

Chapter 5   Healing To and From Animals

Chapter 6   Disaster & Trauma Work

CONNECTING WITH GUIDANCE

Chapter 7   Development of the Healer

CONNECTING WITH NATIVE PEOPLE

Chapter 8   Healing Around the World

INTRODUCTION

Healing Stories is dedicated to the Spirits and people who have shared their Light for others to follow. To them I offer my appreciation and blessings in helping to create this book. May these stories bring a smile or tear, lighten your load, ease your pain, show a new direction, or offer new insights. I am enriched by our contact as we share the path as healers.

This book is about receiving, giving, teaching, and learning energy-based healing. The three parts are: Connecting with Hands and Heart, Connecting with Guidance, and Connecting with Native People. Using the medium of story telling, one is taken dramatically into the lived experience of the participants. Different parts will speak to different people. However, much can be learned about the new world of energy based-healing that is actually based on ancient teachings. All the stories are based on real experiences in receiving, giving, teaching, and learning Healing Touch and Energetic Healing. In some cases the names and circumstances have been changed to protect identity and privacy.

Theses stories are primarily written to and for the Healing Touch and Energetic Healing communities, since they are derived from the practice of these two energy modalities. However, they can be read by anyone interested in exploring the rich dimensions of healing. These stories are intended to inspire and to help promote a deeper understanding of the mysteries of life.

The decision was made to do this book in the early 1990's after years of teaching energy-based healing worldwide. I was struck with the magnificent tapestry of healing experiences that students reported to me. I knew their stories needed to be told. I knew it was time for me to put down my stories as well.

Welcome to the world of healing stories. Sharing stories can teach us new ways to connect energetically and show us new aspects of healing. It is my hope that this book helps enrich your healing journey.

Love,
     Light,
        Laughter,

Mary Jo Bulbrook
Carrboro, North Carolina
January 2000

STORY ABOUT THE COVER

Inspiration from White Eagle
(Geelong, Victoria, Australia, March 1996)

An Indian appeared to me the morning of my Healing Touch workshop in Geelong in 1996 and said he wanted to speak through me. I told him that I didn't have time and besides, we do not channel in Healing Touch! He repeated his message. As I prepared to start the workshop, he spoke again instructing me to tell my friend what he said. I followed his instructions. My friend replied, "I was wondering when he would show up. That has to be White Eagle." He is one of her guides. I asked her to write what I said if I went into trance as I wouldn't remember afterwards. At the end of the morning meditation, White Eagle came and gave the Inspiration that appears on the cover of the book.

Connecting with the Artist
(Geelong, Victoria, Australia, March 1997)

I was looking for over a year to find a way to share the inspiration. One day while I was teaching again in Geelong, Victoria in Australia at the same place that I received the White Eagle message, my friends Janeece and Colin Kelsall, who have a magazine called *Spiritual Links,* handed me the March '97 edition with the Southern Cross Landscape Temple on the cover. As I viewed the drawing and felt the energy, I knew that White Eagle's words needed to be connected to the drawing. I was taken to meet artist, Charles Bartlett. We made arrangements that day to put our contributions together. Charles gave me the original drawing and it has a place of honor in my home in North Carolina.

Southern Cross Landscape Temple
(Charles Bartlett, Pencil and Ink, 1995)

I had been connected with a group of dedicated earth workers, who had been meeting and meditating on the five mountain points in Victoria of the southern landscape temple, at certain times over a one hundred day period in accordance with information received by spirit. These points are Mt. Buninyong in the West, Mt. Macedon in the North, Mt. Dandenong in the East, the You Yangs in the South and the fifth point being Cobbledicks Ford in the southeast. These points are a mirror image of the stars comprising the Southern Cross Constellation. This drawing, is an attempt at showing the vision I was given of the Southern Cross Landscape Temple and its inherent powers, while involved in one of the linking meditations.

Connections across the World

Spirit again linked people to spread their message. We are proud and honored to pass this work on to you and share in the energy of the spiritual drawing and spiritual words. May they bring as much joy and pleasure to you as they have to us.

Mary Jo Bulbrook
Charles Bartlett
Janeece & Colin Kelsall

EDITOR'S NOTE

In August, 1999 I attended a HT Level III A class in Durham, NC and met Mary Jo (the course instructor) for the first time. One day over lunch she asked if I would be interested in working with her on a collection of healing stories. I was intrigued with the idea, but if Mary Jo had asked me in advance to help produce a 300-page book in three months, I would have said it was impossible. The form and content of this book evolved from a simple collection of stories into a rich tapestry of healing partnerships around the world. As we got involved in the process I was reminded once again that faith can produce miracles. Mary Jo and I received guidance every step of the way. Stories came pouring in. And for the most part, we tried to retain the "voice" of each contributor and allow each person to tell their story in their own words. I am very grateful to all the folks who contributed to this project. Seeing the kind of healing work people are doing all over the world touched and inspired me. In sharing our stories we not only learn about who we are, but we also discover who we can become by connecting with our heart and hands in the work of healing.

Peace,

Dan Trollinger

NOTES ON THE PHOTOGRAPH SECTION

Page #1   Connections with Mother Mary
Excerpt from Mary's first message to me January 8, 1993 to share with the world. Statue of Mother Mary from a monastery outside Perth, Western Australia where I was called to take the first tour to Australia and assist orphaned Aborigine spirits in making their transition. Photograph of the rainbow image of the Virgin Mary that appeared on December 17, 1996 on a financial building in Clearwater, Florida. Madonna of the Window appeared a few days after Barbara Harris asked for a sign to share her conversations with Mary.

Page #2   Journey to the Light — Pyramid Labyrinth
The design of the Labyrinth was channeled to me January 1, 1997. Focus includes four directions and Archangels (Uriel, East – Emotion; Gabriel, South – Physical; Raphael, West – Mind; Michael, North – Spirit). The seven chakras and seven layers of the auric field are represented. Rose and Joe Pere are walking the Labyrinth in Cincinnati, Ohio while on the 1997 tour. A group walks the Labyrinth in Hawaii during a retreat.

Page #3   Energy Manifestations
Although not visible to the naked eye, these energy manifestations were captured on film. Images show the Light of Spirit connections around people and in caves.

Page #4   Clinical Pictures — Teaching Around the World
Includes visual picture of cancer of the head, aura drawings from Roger Weinstein on a client with AIDS/HIV; an aura drawing by Mary Jo done September 22, 1993 showing a heart-centered person; a visualization of the expanded Core Star illustrating the return to health and sharing our inner light (illustrated by Katherine Kubel to show the emanating Light).

Page #5   Aura Pictures of Littleton, Colorado
These drawings come from Janna Moll and others in her work to heal those affected by the Littleton, CO shooting crisis. On April 20, 1999 waves of hate, fear, and panic spread throughout the world. Two aura drawings done on April 22 illustrate the effect on a male near the pipebombs and a female who heard the terror and felt the pain of lost friends. The center photo is of the healing that took place from the Earth Healing Technique channeled to Sally Clements. Janna led a group healing on site to clear the land of residual energy manifestations. Finally, three drawings done by those who held the energy for Janna on site while the healing was performed. All show a vortex of energy over the area that then radiated outward.

Page #6   Animal Healers and Healing

Logo of HT for Animals, Carol Komitor, and Bogard, Carol's beloved dog healer. Annis Parker, Director of Natural Health for Animals of HTP, spirit healers Ginger and Chaney Bulbrook, Paul Forman healing a kangaroo and holding the owl that I did a healing on. Leslie White feeling the energy of a camel while on tour in Australia. Donna holding a thorny lizard in Australia. Feeding a South African bird. Healing horses in Ohio, New Zealand, and Australia.

Page #7   Land Healings

Connecting with trees, in Hawaii, Australia, and New Zealand. Healing on Stone Mountain led by Rose Pere on tour in 1997. Hawaiian site of earth cross where trapped spirits who committed suicide were held as I was teaching the group to read earth signs.

Page #8   The Healing Touch Partnerships Family

The home of NC Center for Healing Touch. Key faculty: Mary Jo Bulbrook, Donna Duff, Cathy Mack, Gayla Wood. Staff: Bill (Business Manager) and Jim Bulbrook (Webmaster). Bernie Clarke, International Coordinator of EH Program and Senior Wellness; Liz Duff, Canadian Partner; Cindy Ross, South African Partner; Hug Bear for Healing; Anne Boyd and EH Angel; the Australia Partner, Janeece and Colin Kelsall of *Spiritual Links* Magazine; Cath Webber Martin, Dimensional and Spiritual Healing; Warwick Hain, Craig and Sue Pattinson of New South Wales; Reo Jameson, the past NZ Partner; Annis Parker, NZ, International Coordinator of HTP and Director and Founder of Natural Health for Animals; Carol Komitor and Janna Moll of HT for Animals; Native healers showing the family team: Rose Pere, Maori Tohuna, New Zealand; Bob Randall, Aborigine of Central Australia.

Page #9   Connections with Virginia Satir

Personal letter to me from Virginia on June 4, 1976. John Thie, creator of Touch for Health, colleague and friend with Virginia; Gordon Stokes, friend and past international director of TFH is included. Virginia with world famous healer Olga Worrell in the early 1970's. Some members of Avanta Network, Virginia's organization. I organized the first international training for Avanta Network in the 1980's and was on the original Board of Directors to help shape that organization.

Page #10   Central Australia: Connections with the Aborgines
Traveling and working with the Aborigines and Bob Randall. Signing of
the Aboriginal/Healing Touch Partnerships agreement. Healing Hands,
original art commissioned from Maxine Fumagalli, Denmark, Western
Australia, 1996.

Page #11   Aborigine Healing Touch Partnerships
Uluru (Ayers Rock), Sacred Site of the Aborigines, and Bob Randall's
people of Pitjantjatjara tribe.

Page #12   New Zealand: Tour Experiences and Maori Teachings
Our beloved group in Hawkes Bay, Rose Pere and Reo Jameson, inside a
Marae. Hostess group waving good-bye in the airport in the North Island.
In Nelson, a visit by the Dali Lama is marked by a planting at a historical
site where we held our classes.

Page #13   New Zealand: Tour Experiences
Includes the first HT teachers of NZ trained by Janet Mentgen and Mary Jo
Bulbrook. Donna Duff on site with Maori totem pole. Annis Parker,
Christchurch and Trish Lynch from Nelson. Nancy Stonack from the USA
in NZ on tour, receiving autograph copy of Rose Pere's book *Te Wheke*
during one of her teachings. Rose and Mary Jo doing the hungi.

Page #14   The South African Experience
The Heritage Stone in an iron box that spoke to Credo through me. An
elephant face appeared to me in a dream calling me to South Africa.
Pictures of animals in Skukuza, South Africa. The zebra, a sacred African
animal symbolizing the black and white coming together, also appeared in
a dream calling me there. Throwing of the Bones by African Sangoma, a
member of the Traditional Healers' Association. HT leadership South
Africa group.

Page #15   Partnerships in Ancient Healing: 1997 Tour
Aborigine Way of clearing the land. Connecting on Stone Mountain. Rose
Pere healing Gerry Mitchell. Presentation at the International Council of
Nurses 21st Quadrennial Congress. Board members of the International
Society for the Study of Subtle Energy and Energy Medicine during a sing-
a-long in Boulder, CO.

Page #16   Sunsets
Arranged by Daughter of Sunsets, the Indian name given to Mary Jo.

May I Speak my Truth,
May I Hear my Truth,
May I Live my Truth,

Ever guided by the Divine.
To Clear out the Past,
To Provide the Way
For a New Future
Filled with
Peace, Hope,
Joy and Love.

With Mutual Respect
For Each Other, and May this
Be Known with
Clarity, Sureness and Power.

That I May Deal
With all I need to,
As I Walk
This Path.

White Eagle
through MJB

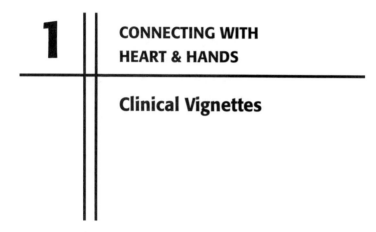

1 CONNECTING WITH HEART & HANDS

Clinical Vignettes

Speaking, Giving, and Being at Peace

It is now almost 12 years since Colleen and I have been together in her healing sessions. In her latest e-mail to me, across the electronic songlines, she shares an update of how the work we did before continues to shape her life today.

Colleen writes: "I remember the wonderful piece of advice you gave me during my healing. I put it in front of me when I need to.

You said, 'Colleen, Speak Your Peace . . . Give Your Peace . . . and Be at Peace.' This is for the moments when I want to put cotton balls in my ears to block out sounds that fill me with anger. I have learned to use these words to move through difficult times."

The work that Colleen and I shared in the healing contact continues to serve not only her in her difficult times, but others as the information has been passed on. Anger, hurt, rage, and disappointment wreck havoc in our lives causing damage to the energy system. In order to be in health, we must rid the energy system of the impact of events, and experiences that have left behind their mark. The subtle influence of our energy over time, can produce not so subtle experiences that changes our lives forever.

Colleen Kelly   *Mary Jo Bulbrook*
St. John's, Newfoundland, Canada   *Carrboro, North Carolina*

A Visual Experience

I have been practicing Healing Touch since 1994, a Certified Healing Touch Practitioner since 1996, and a Certified Healing Touch Instructor since 1998. I have found the stories of intuition and clairvoyance interesting, but beyond my range of experience or possibilities. In the last several years I have studied Energetic Healing with Dr. Bulbrook and began teaching the Energetic Healing program in 1999. It has been a "stretching" experience. I want to share one of many experiences that happen now with increasing frequency that would have seemed impossible to me previously.

A client (HT student) came to my office for supportive help after having just broken off a "harmful relationship." She reported feeling very stressed about this situation. Her chakras and field were open which surprised her. When I had her think of the relationship, all the chakras became compromised, especially the third chakra. The field (aura), Core Star and Hara were not affected. Chelation was done. While I was gently holding her face, I saw energetic hearts radiating off the bottom of her field. Pain Drain was done over third chakra and during the fill phase as clear as day, I *saw* a large Bow sitting on the 7th layer of the field. It was a "happy" bow. Etheric Unruffling and 6th and 7th layer closure were done. When I completed treatment she immediately opened her eyes and said, "I feel finished." When she thought of the relationship after we completed the healing session her chakras maintained an open state. I shared with her what I saw. She immediately related that it made sense to her and confirmed for her that she had made the right decision. She had been having dreams of all kinds of "celebration cakes" since she had ended the relationship. A "happy bow" and hearts radiating from her field represented to her that she was on the right track for what she needed to do.

The point of the story is not so much any specific treatment but rather the visualization of hearts and happy bow that was an observation reflecting and confirming something meaningful to the client. This kind of information is available to us in many subtle ways. *My experiences have grown in direct proportion to my willingness to be open to the possibilities without attachment to any specific experience occurring.*

The nurturance of being open to the possibilities evolved from my work with Dr. Bulbrook. She would so often ask me: "What do you see? What do you sense? What color is there? What message are you hearing or experiencing?" I had much resistance at first because I held the belief that "I don't see and sense things." I was challenged to draw and color what an experience seemed like and began to be surprised that things would come seemingly from "nowhere." As I began to allow myself the possibility of tuning in and receiving useful information, it began to happen more. I pass this on for you to know that extraordinary experiences happen to ordinary folks who are open to the possibilities.

Deny Brown
Richmond, Virginia

Energy is Amazing

There have been more times that I can remember during my ten year career with energy work that I have repeatedly been able, with the assistance of spirit, to shift and decrease or clear pain, ease tension, calm anxiety, promote healing with wounds and increase health and a sense of well being. As skeptical as I was originally, and occasionally still am, the end results continue to amaze me and those I have worked with again and again. The words I hear most often are, "That is amazing." And it is!

While teaching a HT class demonstrating the Chakra Connection, students and I discovered our various intuitive abilities. While I was assessing the energy field connection between chakras kinesthetically, one student acknowledged she could *sense* when the connection was made. Another women *saw* the connection being made and said, "I always thought there was something wrong with my eyes!" I said, "Your eyes are great!" So we acknowledged the intuition of all present and checked the energy system together as we did each step. Confirmation through sharing is an important learning tool and I continue to share that story and pass on all these amazing experiences.

Carol Kinney
San Anselmo, California

A Mystical Experience

John is a 46 year old man who I met when he was hospitalized for surgical removal of part of his lung after being diagnosed with lung cancer. At the time I was a staff registered nurse in the Integrative Health and Medicine department of the hospital in Cincinnati, Ohio. My primary job responsibility was doing Healing Touch everyday with in-patients. I received a request from John for Healing Touch. We had one session prior to his discharge from the hospital. He continued to receive Healing Touch from another practitioner after his discharge and through the local Wellness Community, where Healing Touch is available on a regular basis.

Several months later, John was hospitalized with pneumonia following completion of a course of radiation therapy. He was still receiving chemotherapy. I stopped in to see him at his request. We worked together for the next two days working to strengthen his Hara line, expand his Core Star, open his chakras and clear his energy field. Techniques included both Healing Touch core curriculum such as Magnetic Unruffling, modulation to both lungs and Etheric Vitality plus the Pyramid Balance from the Advanced Practice course taught by Janet Mentgen and the Energy Field Drain and Replenishment taught by Mary Jo Bulbrook in Energetic Healing.

On the third day, due to my schedule, I knew I was not going to have 30-45 minutes to spend with him. I sensed that it was time he was ready to start doing some energy work on his own. He agreed and I gave him a copy of Bulbrook's "Meditation to Balance the Energy System" (from the Energetic Healing program) with a very quick demonstration. This is a wonderful and simple technique to do and to teach clients. The next day his nurse left me a message to be sure to see John. He reported to me that he had done the meditation during the night and proceeded to describe to me what I would call a mystical experience—a profound experience of the presence of God.

John said he saw his aura. The whole experience excited him but also scared him. He said he'd never prayed like that before. John found himself able to feel the energy flow and found that he was putting his hands wherever he thought he needed healing. He also commented that it occurred to him that maybe he is being called to do this work, not right now because he needs to focus on getting well, but down the road. It was good to hear him planning for the future.

As a high school teacher, John could bring the work to a whole new audience some day. John wrote about his experience in his journal and six months later he has returned to teaching. He describes the experience to this day as something he'll never forget.

Mary M. Duennes
Cincinnati, Ohio

Eliminating Tooth Pain

My first experience with Healing Touch was when I attended a Level I class in November 1996. I started the two day course not quite sure what to expect. Over those two days I worked on other people and also had a number of other people work on me.

I had a root canal filling done on one of my back teeth in January of 1996. Following that I had a jaw problem, which caused excruciating pain. I could not open my jaw other than to drink out of a straw. I could only manage to eat soup or something I could slide into my mouth and swallow as I could not move my jaw sideways and could not chew at all. I ended up going to a Chiropractor, hoping he could do cranial or TMJ work. He massaged muscles and it was a little better but did not last. After four visits, I went to an Osteopath in another center. He also helped, but after three visits it was just the same and it kept returning. No one seemed to be able to correct it to last.

I started and finished the Healing Touch class not even thinking of my jaw. I was resigned to the way it was by then. I was always aware of being careful of eating as I could not even bite through a banana. When I left the course and while driving home I realized my jaw was not sore. I kept waiting for the pain and discomfort to return. It never did and it has been A-1 ever since.

This made me realize some powerful work had gone on at the Healing Touch class and that I would complete my training so that I could do the same for others.

Margaret Clare Robertson
Gisborne, New Zealand

Preventing the Need for Surgery

On January 15, 1997 while walking on grass beside the pavement my heel dropped into a hole and twisted. I knew I had broken my ankle. I got myself home, iced it before going to the doctor. He arranged for me to have an x-ray. On returning to his rooms and showing him the x-ray, he declared he could not attempt to do anything himself as it was a transverse fracture of the tip of the malleolus, with separation and displacement of the loose piece of bone. Also the x-ray showed varus tilt of the talus. The medical and posterior malleoli appeared intact, but I would need to see a surgeon who would operate and insert a pin to attach the separated piece of bone back in position. The appointment was scheduled for the next day.

As I lay in my bed that night after being told this news, I decided I was not having any operations or pins. I started energy work, Unruffling and raking the aura (energy field) around my ankle. I then extended the Unruffling as far out from my ankle as my reach would allow. I followed with Ultrasound and finished with a little Laser and then just held the ankle for probably six minutes. All the time I worked, I was talking to my body and my cells, telling them what I wanted them to do. Namely, to realign themselves using their original programming they used before my birth and at the time of my birth. In other words, to recreate themselves in perfection as they had done in utero. I talked to my body until I fell asleep and requested that by morning my ankle would be aligned perfectly.

When I visited the specialist and he looked at my x-ray he confirmed the doctor's comments. It would need an operation and a pin. He had not seen a break quite like it before. However, he said for his own satisfaction he would have it x-rayed again to see how it was sitting right then. I went and had the x-ray. When I returned and he looked at it and said, "Wow, have you looked at this?" I said, "No." He said, "Well I think you'd better for it is perfect and I will be able to plaster it, and it will go on healing OK." He actually said, "That's incredible it's sitting perfectly!"

I totally believe my work made the difference. Each time after when I felt pain I would Ultrasound the ankle for six minutes and the pain would be gone. When I went to the physiotherapist six weeks later, after the plaster came off, I took my two x-rays. On looking at them he said a lot of healing has already gone on in this recent one. I said that's not recent it was taken the next day. He said it couldn't be, it must be in the last day or two, because a heap of healing had already taken place. It could not do that in one day. He was Turkish and it was hard for me to make him understand it was in fact taken the following day, he still thinks it was taken six weeks after the injury.

I was delighted when I realized what this meant. I totally believe the work I did with the energy field surrounding my ankle, within my ankle, and within my mind made the difference between needing surgery and not needing surgery.

Margaret Clare Robertson
Gisborne, New Zealand

Pain Drain

A previous client called for an appointment to see if I could help her with chronic jaw pain of several months duration only partially relieved with pain medication. She had a history of an abscessed tooth that had been treated with antibiotics. Follow up x-rays and evaluations were normal, yet she had persistent pain. She was dismissed by an oral surgeon who said, "You shouldn't have pain now because tests are clear." I used the Pain Drain on the jaw area and felt a heavy hot, thick substance (that I would describe "like hot glue") flow out of my palm for about ten minutes. After the Pain Drain stopped and I energized the area, she reported she no longer felt any pain. In follow-up she has not had a reoccurrence. The interesting thing about this session was her statement at end of session: "I don't know what you did but for awhile I felt like 'hot glue' was pouring out of my ear." I had not told her what it had felt like to me.

This summer my daughter provided me with two dramatic experiences with Unruffling and Pain Drain. These were the primary treatments around surgery support for correction of fractured deviated septum in her nose and some extensive gum surgery. Both of which are usually accompanied by swelling and bruising. At times these symptoms would be quite extensive as well as pain postoperatively. In both situations I mostly did Unruffling and then Pain Drains every few hours. With each successive drain the release decreased. At her 24 hour post-op check up she had no bruising from either procedure, required minimal pain medication and very little swelling (and that was released quickly with the drains).

Deny Brown
Richmond, Virginia

Kasha and the Angel's Visit

I am a psychiatric home health nurse who was recently asked by my supervisor to case manage a medical/surgical patient for another nurse who was leaving the agency. I went to visit Kasha, a little Russian lady in her 80's who had an 18 year old cat, Meisa, who was her "best friend." After I performed my medical/surgical assessment, Kasha was anxious for me to leave, stating that she didn't need any more health care people intruding on her. I validated her feelings, and wanting to respect her right to be alone. As I was gathering my nursing bag to get ready to leave, I heard my angel telling me to stay.

So I just sat there on her sofa, feeling rather uncomfortable about not respecting her wish. The silence seemed interminable when at last she looked over at me and began to tell me how distraught she was about not sleeping very well for several months. I felt prompted to tell her that I do Healing Touch and I was starting to explain when she said, "Well, you know, I've always been interested in Yoga and that sort of thing, so go ahead." As she sat in her recliner, I maneuvered around her doing Magnetic Unruffling and Mind Clearing while her cat, Meisa, sat nestled on her breast. Interestingly, I looked up during the treatment and on her wall before me was a precious drawing of Jesus holding a lamb in the very same position. When I was done, Kasha told me that she never felt such peace before and that God sent me to her.

She proceeded to tell me the story of the painting of Jesus and the lamb. She said that she was middle-aged and feeling desperate and alone when this black and white picture blew across the sidewalk and landed at her feet. She said that she took it home and felt led to color in a beautiful golden aura around Jesus and the lamb. She casually said, "I just felt the energy in the picture." Then, as I was sitting across from her (listening to the story of her life and including how she fled the Communists as a young child), she looked at me and said very matter of factly, "You have a very big angel over your left shoulder. I can see him. He's very beautiful, and young, about 20 years old and has long hair. He loves you so much! And I don't know why, but he has his finger up to his lips as if he's saying 'sssshhhhh.'"

I was awestruck! I felt tears swelling up in my eyes and such a heart connection with this precious lady. What a gift Kasha has been to me! I believe that my angel was saying "sssshhh" to always remind me to listen for guidance about how to open my heart to love in every encounter. And by the way, Kasha has been sleeping very well since the Healing Touch.

Kathleen Letke
Chapel Hill, North Carolina

Changing the Course of Leanne's Life

Leanne is a three year old beautiful soul suffering from severe epilepsy. She doesn't walk or talk. When she came to me as a client, she had frequent small and large seizures every day and constant grinding of her teeth. The medical world had given up on her and told the parents to look elsewhere as they did all they knew to do. I believe the way the parents came across my business card was Divine Intervention. On the day they were told to look for alternatives to help their daughter, the father went to the letterbox outside his home and found my card on the driveway. We have no idea how it got there!

I have seen Leanne in the first couple of months weekly and at the moment every fortnight. The grinding of the teeth has completely gone! To me, it is as if her soul has accepted her journey. The frequency and severity of seizures has lessened significantly. The parents do the Chakra Connection on her every day. It is the only time Leanne allows them to touch and hold her head without a fight. Leanne has become a smiling, happy child, who has a better concentration span and is now willing to try to stand with special ankle supports. Healing Touch changed the course of her life, and mine as well.

Marijke Klumpers
Havelock North, New Zealand

Looking into the Eyes of a Healer

My own eyes widen as I gaze into the eyes of a healer. I am first drawn to the deep pools of wisdom which gaze lovingly back into my own. In the depths of those eyes there is knowledge of ego, but ego kept in check by the universal understanding that all healing is a gift between God and the soul in wait. Then I see the mental body bright, intuitive, knowing, but waiting for the other to see their knowingness and accept in totality their grace. Tiny lines surround their physical eyes, eyes filled with compassion and caring. They too have experienced pain, and respect in turn the pain of the one they seek to help. The brightness of their physical eyes sparkle with spirit, for they know oneness, peace, harmony, blessings. Indeed, they know God. To all of us, with heartfelt gratitude may we heal ourselves as we gaze into our mirrors. Inspired by a shared moment with Mary Jo—a heart healing.

Lori Protzman
Aeia, Hawaii

Intent
It is with "intent" that you
touch the human soul.
It is with compassion that you
touch and that you hold.
It is with a listening ear that you
hear another's heart.
It is in the "being" that you
feel what might impart.
Bring your focus to the spirit
that lies beneath your hands.
Allow that part of you to know
what the head can't understand.
In the space and in the moment
sacred time is spent,
As love transcends the essence
what is called "intent."

Deborah Larrimore
Winston-Salem, North Carolina

Keep on Dancing
I have been an avid Israeli dancer for a number of years in that I
would dance 2 1/2 hours 1-2 times a week. In the 15 minute ride home
after dance class, I would become so stiff that when I would get out
of the car, I was moving like someone 110 years old. After taking
Level I Healing Touch, I began to do self Chakra Connection at least
once or twice a week with no particular goal in mind except self
balancing. About six weeks into this new practice I was aware that
I no longer became stiff on the ride home from dance class. This year
I expanded my dance experience to include intense four-day dance
camps where we literally dance 6-12 hours a day. Needless to say by
2:00 a.m. we could hardly move and even our toes hurt. My
roommate had taken an introductory class in HT from me and was
used to using the Pain Drain with relief, but this was not sufficient for
dance camp. The first night she was unable to sleep due to painful
legs even with elevating them and taking extra strength tylenol. The
second day she came in when I was doing self Chakra Connection so
I invited her to follow along with me. She fell asleep easily without

pain though we had danced twice as long that day. I'd like to pass on a prescription for dance camp: Chakra Connection and Pain Drain to the toes before each nap, and then dance to your heart's content.

Deny Brown
Richmond, Virginia

Faith and Healing

An 80 year old man who lost his wife six months ago was in the hospital. He has a small tumor in the back, is a long time recovering alcoholic and suffers from bouts of alcoholic depression. A month or so ago, I worked on some painful areas in his back doing energy work, as well as counseling on and off over the last year. On this particular day he said he wished he could have the faith that I had. I asked him if he really wanted it and where would it be in his body if he had it. He pointed to his forehead (at the area of the third eye). I immediately laid one hand over his third eye and one behind the back of his head and prayed for the faith he asked for. I held the hands there about 30 seconds, let go, and his face was beaming.

Agnes Sanford said, "Pray like it's happening and it will." I am already changing, becoming more bold to do things like this without fear or hesitation. Faith is openness. As I am open, I can help others to open as well. Perhaps we are really more tied together than we realize. If we live what we believe, we model this for others. Faith is openness—being led into the unknown by the One we know.

The Reverend Mark Bigley
Arlington, Texas

Comic Alignment

I picked John, my 18 year old son, up at the airport for the two hour trip back to the house. I was really excited about having uninter-rupted time to tell him about all I was learning in Healing Touch. I talked about pendulums, chakras, auras, and energy level. He patiently listened and I was surprised the he only rolled his eyes once!

As we were driving I hit a pot hole and commented that I needed to get new shocks. "Well Mom," my son smugly said. "Maybe you should take the car in for a chakra alignment!"

Jean Marie Givens-Myers
Williamsburg, Virginia

The Rule Keeper

Having gotten to HT Level IIIA, my mind was cluttered with the "rules" of each procedure. I often had my workbook open to ensure during the procedures "right." Since I was a professional rule keeper, I wondered if I would ever get it right. On the third day, I expressed this to Mary Jo in class. The message through her guidance was:

I'm doing the best I can. I surrender. Show me the way.

After this message, there was a spinning on the top of my head like a helicopter propeller. At the same time I felt my head and face fill with a very powerful energy connecting me to the Divine Source. How blessed I felt!

Helen Boyd
Glen Allen, Virginia

Impacting the Symptoms of Multiple Sclerosis

Early in my HT career, I was called to see a women with Multiple Sclerosis. She was in her early thirties, had been a very active and successful business woman. Now, in a years time, she was bed bound, unable to care for herself except through her thoughts and words. She often was in extreme discomfort with spasms in her extremities and had no control of her limbs. Her husband and children did their best to care for her, but there were many challenges for all. Her mother often visited and was her main caregiver. Occasionally, a local home health agency also visited. M never complained and was grateful for any assistance. She wanted most to be able to care for her family in any way she could, to feel more at ease and be able to rest. Her aunt had taught her to open her chakras in her mind and she regularly practiced this activity. I was asked to aid in her comfort with energy work. M was very accepting of this work and loved to have me come.

During the two years we worked together, M was very brave. With her mind she kept up with all the family activities of her husband and children. Often when I came she would be in severe spasms. I used the Chakra Connection, Magnetic Unruffling, and the Chakra Spread to help her relax. When I left M would be sleeping or dozing. I taught her mother and M to do the self Chakra Connection. M would do the Chakra Connection in her mind and often upon my arrival, much to my surprise, her centers would be open. I would say to her, "Of all the clients I see, I almost always find your chakras open. How do you do that M?" Then we would laugh and we would repeat this each visit. I was in awe of how she could mentally open her energy centers each visit. M gave me a beautiful silver pin in the shape of a hand with a heart shaped rose quartz in its center. I wear it often while teaching. It is a great reminder of our connection and how Healing Touch helps even when there seems to be so few solutions to a client's discomfort.

Carol Kinney
San Anselmo, California

Cardiac Care

Mrs. A came to see me complaining of headache, neck pain, and numbness in her hands for about eight months and some chest discomfort. She is 62 years old and lives alone. Her medical history includes heart bypass surgery, a laminectomy (L 4-5), knee replacement, diabetes, hypertension, hypothyroidism, and dye from mylograms that never dissipated. She has a cardiologist and an internist. She is on several medications.

During the first session, I used the Spiral Meditation, Chakra Connection, and Magnetic Unruffling. At one point the client opened her eyes and said, "I can't believe this my hands are not numb anymore I can feel!" I then worked on her back and neck (Pain Drain, Ultrasound, Hopi Back Technique). Intuitively, I did Etheric Unruffling next, I then discovered an energy leak over her heart. I then sealed the leak, modulated energy there, and proceeded to close the Spiral. The client sat up and was in tears. She said she couldn't remember the last time she felt that good.

Several months later she shared with me what really happened. Two weeks before she saw me originally, she had suffered another heart attack. She returned to her doctor a couple of weeks after her Healing Touch treatment and told him her chest pain was now gone. She told the doctor her healer felt a leak over her heart and the doctor said he heard her mitral valve leaking at her last visit. The doctor examined her, he told her that the audible leak he had heard was gone. He did another EKG and could not find the cardiac damage that had been previously documented. My client has felt well for one year now.

Debbie Karl
Clinton, NY

My Difficulties
My father said it was all in my head (i.e. my imagination).
Edith Fiore would say it's in my attached entities.
Gary Zukav would say it's in my choices.
Valerie Hunt would say it's all in my mind field.
The Catholics would say it's my lack of belief in JC.
Linda Goodman would say it's in my planetary line-up.
Hannah Kroger and Hulda Clark would say it's in my parasites.
Caroline Myss would say it's in my biography.
Larry Dossey would say it's in my words.
A yogi would say it's my karma.
Jung — my shadow. Freud — my neuroses, Jampolski — my fears.
Energy workers — my low vibratory rate.
Rolfers — my armoring. Sondra Ray — improper breathing.
Lauren Artress and Scott Peck would know I got off the beaten path.
Markides — my inability to travel between dimensions.
Chopra — one or more of at least seven reasons.
A shaman would recommend retrieving the lost parts of my soul.
Alice Bailey — my lack of initiation. Louise Hay — my affirmations.
Euclid — my geometry is not sacred.

Here I believed Robert Anthony when he said, "We're all whole, complete and perfect." But I have just reeled off a list of some pretty prestigious names that dispute that whole idea. Indeed, we probably need to be fixed.

Jane Hock
Houston, Texas

Expelling Energy
One afternoon while attending my HT Level II class, the room was quiet in a spiritual space. The teacher announced for the healees to get on their tables. Mood set, lights lowered, room quieter than quiet, as my partner slide up on the table, a large amount of flatus was expelled. Everyone in the room just turned around and looked my way. While trying to keep the mood and my composure, I began with Unruffling, hand over hand. I thought that was a good choice at the time and taught another way of expelling energy.

Carol Jordan
Raleigh, North Carolina

Head of the Class

It doesn't take long in the role of instructor to experience the importance of what you say because of students tendency to respond in a very literal way. In a recent HT Level I class I had given instructions before voice guiding the chakra connection, where I asked that the students who were on the table to have their head at the end of the table that was closest to the blackboard. (Having students all in same direction facilitates being able to see if the students doing the technique are able to follow your directions.) Several of the students were not following that request so as a general reminder without singling anyone out I stated, " All heads to the blackboard." The students lying down sat up to face the blackboard, and all the remaining students who were standing waiting to give the technique also did a military about face towards the blackboard. A sense of humor helps in this work. When I could stop laughing at what I had inadvertently created, I was able to state to the class what I actually wanted them to do.

Deny Brown
Richmond, Virginia

Source of Healing

A friend asked me to work on her, but I was feeling so frazzled that week that I decided to put her off for another week. The next morning in my meditation I was told that she needed me now and that I should work on her. So I called her immediately and scheduled her for sooner. The morning she was to come, I did my usual preparation including meditating, but it was the first time that I couldn't get my chakras to open. I started to panic and thought I'd have to tell her that I couldn't work on her when she came. Then I heard a voice tell me, "You're not the one who opens your chakras or does the healing. Let go now." Much to my surprise I did! In an instant all my chakras were open and then rainbow colors surrounded me and my client (before she arrived). I felt very peaceful and very humble and I realized that my ego can get in the way both by thinking, "I'm doing something," or by thinking, "I'm not good enough to do it." I was told that my intent and my "yes" were good enough and that they would work there in my brokenness. In fact, I experienced a very special healing during the session with my client and my client later told me it was her most profound healing so far.

The healing in me was that I saw myself in my first Communion dress as a seven year old little girl. I was so pure and so in touch with spirit. I had been made fun of for being "too holy" by my peers and so I had become afraid and lost my connection. In just one moment, I reintegrated that precious seven year old girl back inside of me. The tears of joy just flowed!

Kathleen Letke
Chapel Hill, North Carolina

Two Sides of the Same Story

Client: *"Mary, I believe that I have been healed. I'm no longer on oxygen, taking 3/4's of my pills and my friends and family say I look 10 years younger. Well, I DO feel much better and my color is better but you KNOW, everyone always says I look so good. I've been in the hospital twice and spent lots of time in recovery, but my new doctor insisted on these measures. I certainly am happy to give up pills. The hardest thing is going off prednisone. I miss you. Since you have played such a big part in keeping me going, I wanted you to know that the man up stairs has been working all along. It is incredible!"*

Practitioner: I'm forwarding this e-mail (above) that came today from my beloved Evergreen Hospice client, who I treated as my first hospice client as a HT volunteer in August 1995. I continued to see her weekly for a year and a half, by which time, she had flunked Hospice 101 and was discharged to medicare. Ann then paid for my services weekly until July 1999 when I moved out of state. She was the subject of my Healing Touch case study. Within a week after my departure, she made the huge decision to leave the retirement center she hated, and move over to the Olympic peninsula to be nearer her daughter and grandchildren. In doing so, she had to give up her last connection to her old life, and her long term doctors. She jumped, and the proverbial net appeared. She nearly died of pneumonia the week after she moved. Her new doctors, looking at her as a new patient, had the courage to start cutting back her medications. She was too ill to protest, and survived. A month later, her heart slowed to 25 beats a minute. She called 911, was hospitalized, given a pacemaker, and found to have serious potassium imbalance. The pacemaker was removed. She was shown once again, that she could survive. Since our first meeting, I have seen Ann, then 56, as a vibrant, beautiful person; one who suffers not so much from the physical ailments that have plagued her, but from a soul sickness. I believe somewhere in the upheaval of mid-life, she had lost track of her reason for living.

In 1994, shortly after Ann was declared "terminal" with incurable respiratory and mitral valve disease, her husband of 30 years was diagnosed with cancer and proceeded to die within a year of the diagnosis. I entered her life on the one year anniversary of his death, when she was already six-months over her own estimated death date. Because she was one of those obedient, "good" patients, she even felt like a failure because she had failed to die when the doctors had predicted! We have learned so much from each other. It has been an honor and a joy to be a part of her journey. We owe our connection to Healing Touch—and to the Hospice program that had the courage to initiate the Compassionate Touch volunteer program that brought us together.

Mary Ellis
Olympia, Washington

Pain-Free for the First Time in Years

I co-created a HT clinic four years ago to offer HT healers the opportunity to come and practice and receive HT for themselves. We also set the intention and have continued to offer HT and EH to all members of our local community whether they could pay or not. During one of these session, I worked with a grandmother of one of our regular clients who brought her grandmother because of severe back pain. This elderly woman had been told by her doctors, "That she would never be without pain and there was nothing they could do." Rather than argue this point, I offered to work with her. She choose to lie on her side on the massage table making the treatment on her back questionable, since the abdominal position would have been favorable. Grandmother continued her mantra of what the doctors had told her during most of the treatment. I continued to do the treatment. When I was finished she acknowledged some easing of the pain, and thanked me. A day later, I received a phone call from the granddaughter asking me to call her grandmother because, "She would be thrilled to just hear from you." I called her and received the wonderful news that she was pain-free for the first time in years.

Carol Kinney
San Anselmo, California

Healing Touch and Knee Replacement Surgery

Surgery support is a service that I offer with Healing Touch but this case had several unusual aspects that I had not encountered before. This is not a detailed case study but rather a description of happenings that made this an interesting experience. Sue was in her late 40's and had suffered a serious leg injury as a result of an accident almost 25 years ago. Since that time she has had trouble with her left knee and had been resisting having knee replacement surgery for many years. At the time of our first appointment she had knee replacement surgery scheduled for the next day. She had been told because of the old injury and scar tissue build up to expect a particularly difficult recovery. She was told she would need a morphine pump for several days to control pain and would require walking with canes or a walker for some time. During the pre-op session the left leg was very slow to allow the energy to flow. Her hands levitated in the air without physical support and remained that way throughout most of the session. This would occur again in the recovery room and for one additional post-op session. I saw her in recovery room and for the next two days post-op. She was discharged ahead of schedule on post-op day two, without canes and with minimal post-op pain. The morphine pump line had come loose in first 24 hours and they did not restart it as she had not been using it.

On post-op day one while doing HT session in hospital I was directing energy to the left knee from the field, when I observed the left leg begin to raise up off the bed and move slowly and gently as if being put through range of motion exercises. Client was in apparent altered state and said she was not aware of the leg movement during the session. Before I told her what happened I asked her after the session if she was able to move the leg at all which was in a heavy metal support frame. She was unable to move it in conscious state. I also noted that a hematoma near the incision edge disappeared at the end of this session. This same movement happened again during one of her follow up sessions at home. Her recovery went very well and about two months post-op she called to report that she had been so distracted worrying about the knee surgery that she had completely forgotten to mention that she had a history of severe migraines 3-4 times a week since the age of four and she suddenly realized that she had not had one since the pre-op visit. This occurred two years ago and in recent follow up, the client reports that she has had only a few migraines in the last two years and none as severe as what she used to experience on a several times a week basis for over forty years.

Deny Brown
Richmond, Virginia

Chorus of Friends

Diana was dying from a cancerous brain tumor and was experiencing horrific headaches which the pain management team could not seem to help. The staff called me hoping Healing Touch would bring her moments of rest. She was 37, and not happy with the cards she felt she had been dealt. Family and friends were with her around the clock, but would tiptoe in and out so as not to "disturb" her. Their lack of disturbance, disturbed her even more, I observed. She often would pull the sheet over her face in lieu of having to stare at me.

Often when I would come for a treatment session, family would hastily leave, welcoming the chance to escape, yet not abandoning her. In these quiet moments of healing she would share her anger and fear. One day a circle of her best friends were present. One in the group was a local, well known entertainer. She sings of the Hawaiian Islands and her humor captures everyone as she entertains. The singer is a very large Hawaiian woman whose physical presence in itself is a joy.

The love this group of women held for Diana was touching. They were in perfect harmony with her and although saddened by Diana's angry bursts and sarcastic words, they accepted her totally. Around them she glowed and it was this special group of women I taught the chakra spread. As Diana began slipping in and out of consciousness, the group worked feverishly with the energy. It kept them busy and connected them to her. Occasionally she would suddenly sit bolt upright and stare fixedly ahead, agitated and seemingly in pain. We would unruffle her field and they would again begin the chakra spread, each of the four taking turns.

The singer cried softly as she did her round of the spread. Diana suddenly sat up and looked into her eyes and asked sternly, "What are you crying about?" Her friend told her to, "Shut up and go back to heaven, if she wanted to cry she could." Diana smiled at her and then said, "Fine, and by the way I asked God once I enter heaven if

I could make you skinny, and He said, Yes!" The entertainer then
said, "So get out of here and make me skinny. What you waiting for
anyway?"

That was the last Diana spoke. I left the women and told them I
would return later in the day. Several hours later I came back to check
on Diana. I could hear laughter and voices raised in raucous song. I
opened Diana's door. Diana had left shortly after I left her room
earlier. But her spirit seemed everywhere and the joy her friends felt
at her leaving in peace and humor brought them a peace they never
thought they would experience. They continued to lovingly do the
spread as family gathered to say good-bye.

Lori Protzman
Aiea, Hawaii

Changing Belief Systems

I had been working with Jim who is in his 60's and who has been
haunted from a traumatic early childhood that has left him fearful
and very limited in being able to function in this life because no
matter what he tried he couldn't escape his childhood wounds. He
was a professional client in that he was always seeking out the "new
treatment" that would make him be "healed." However, it was
always eluding him and thought to be outside of himself. He had a
tendency to be very dependent on whoever the current provider was,
so it was important to set very clear boundaries and to reinforce the
goal of self-empowerment.

In one recent session he was willing to work with identifying and
changing a belief that was limiting him. He discovered that core
belief to be, "I do not deserve to receive anything good in life." Using
EH techniques I cleared that belief energetically and then anchored
in the new belief that he chose to replace the limiting belief. The
following week he was like a different person. He called to say that
old fears had come up that had always overwhelmed him before and
he decided to see if he could rebalance himself. He was elated to
discover that he had been able to shift the feeling on his own which
was a major milestone change for him. I have seen him for a few
sessions since, and while his progress is in process, his sense of self
and his energy system are clearly stronger. He is beginning to take

steps in his life. I have found Energetic Healing a program that has accelerated my own healing as well as my clients' healing. This why I pursued training to be able to teach this work to others and pass on how to help others heal.

Deny Brown
Richmond, Virginia

Repairing Breast Reconstruction Aftereffects

When I was visiting a friend who had surgery for breast cancer six months earlier, she was telling me about a disturbing symptom that she had. R had gone to the doctor complaining of, "Not feeling like herself." She was having trouble concentrating and did not have the stamina to deal with things like before. Her sense of balance was gone as well. The doctors said she would just need to learn to live with it. I offered to do energy work on her. She agreed although never had anything like this done before. On examining R's field the most striking thing that I noticed was that over the abdomen she did not have an etheric layer. I questioned R about the findings and she related that the doctor had done a breast reconstruction and used tissue over the abdomen. Her belly button was gone!

I rebuilt the entire first layer of the field that supports physical life (etheric layer) by placing my hand over the area slightly above the body about an inch to two inches. It worked like icing a cake. I kept building the layer until it felt nice and full and fluffy. This the best way I can describe it.

R remarked that she felt different and clearer in the head. We worked no longer than about five minutes. She got up and went home. A week later we were together. She remarked that she did not have any of the symptoms that she had reported before and her family and friends commented how different she was.

Once again I became aware of the power in energy work, of doing "little" things that turn out to be not so little! I realize that any time someone has surgery it will be important to check the etheric layer over the treatment site to see if it needs to be rebuilt as well as cleared.

Mary Jo Bulbrook
Carrboro, North Carolina

Spontaneous Hip Recovery

Ed is a 53 year old male with a current complaint that includes pain in bilateral hip joints with an onset in April 1996. He was diagnosed first with greater trochanteric bursitis and treated by steroid injections without success. From 1989-1995 he had cancer of the colon, cancer of the kidney coronary artery disease resulting in triple bypass surgery, pancreatitis, and a gall bladder removed. Ed agreed to be my HT case study. Sessions began on May 30, 1996 and were once per week using energetic techniques only. In June the diagnosis was changed to bilateral avascular necrosis of the femoral neck. For this he underwent decompression surgery to the left hip in an attempt to facilitate bone regeneration. No procedure was done on the right hip except Healing Touch. Ed continued to receive HT treatments for a total of 12 sessions between May 30 and September 26. The results were remarkable! The status of the left hip, which underwent decompression surgery, was 75% healed after only 12 weeks post-op. This procedure usually takes 6-12 months to heal. The right hip, which only received HT was completely healed! The physical status of each leg was also significant. The joint range of motion and muscle strength was preserved in the right hip, which had not been subjected to surgery and was treated by HT!

Joanne G. Dupre
South Dartmouth, Massachusetts

Healer's Prayer

I am here only to be truly helpful.
I am here to represent Him who sent me.
I do not have to worry about what to say or what to do because
    He who sent me will direct me.
I am content to be wherever He wishes,
    knowing He goes there with me.
I will be healed as I let Him teach me to heal.

From *A Course In Miracles*

2 | CONNECTING WITH HEART & HANDS

Family Healing Stories

What Moms Are Made Of
Kisses and laughter in the mornings,
    Joy and importance in the afternoon,
        And love and comfort at night.

The touch of an angel when we need it most,
    The roar of a lion to remind us,
        And the knowledge of a owl to lead us
            In the right direction.

Out of the things they are,
    The most important is,
        They need to be taken care of sometimes
            Like the earth.

Abby Velting (Age 11)
Detroit, Michigan

Merry Christmas, I Love You

Henry had suffered a stroke which left him with a weakness on his right side involving both his arm and leg. His speech was slowed and he had difficulty getting the words out at times. He knew what he wanted to say but sometimes the words just wouldn't come. His reason for coming for Healing Touch was to: "Make my snapper fingers longer, and make my voice better."

As I assessed the chakras. My intuition told me to go back to the heart chakra. It was not in alignment with the others and it had indeed shifted to the right. It was as if it had just slide down the side. I restructured and realigned it to its proper place. I continued with the Chakra Connection.

I saw Henry several more times and his heart chakra remained in place. At our session in November he was very excited to share with me his plan for Christmas. He and his wife had been married for over 40 years. He had never bought her a present, always giving cash with the loving thought, "Go buy yourself what ever you want honey." Now he wanted to buy her the gold nugget on a chain she talked and dreamed about. "Where do I go?" he asked. I gave him directions to the local jewelry store and gave it no than a passing thought in the weeks before Christmas.

Henry came to his Healing Touch session after the holidays beaming. He had gone to he jewelry store, selected, paid for, and wrapped himself the prized gold nugget on a chain. He tenderly placed the small package on his wife's breakfast plate on Christmas morning.

"Merry Christmas, I love you. I know it's been a long time since I told you that."

His dog still doesn't respond to his snapper and some words are still elusive, but my, how his heart is open and in the right place! Healing takes many forms.

Cathy Mack
Garner, North Carolina

Hug Bear for Healing

1. HUG BEAR'S BIRTH

While I was living in Newfoundland, I was separated from my three children for a time due to a number of unavoidable circumstances. I became very concerned that my oldest son was having difficulty. I felt helpless being so far away to help him. I wanted him to know that I was there for him. One day I decided to buy a very large brown teddy bear. My goal was to "hug" the bear and send that "hug" which represented care, comfort, and love to him via the energy lines of our connection that was present through time and space. I nicknamed the bear "Hug Bear" or HB for short. HB is the initials of my son as well.

When I was reunited with my children I told them the story and how important it was to me for them to feel and experience concretely my love. Over the years we have told that story to a number of people.

On day one of my oldest son's friends was in deep trouble and in deep despair over a tragedy that happened to him. I counseled my son and told him his friend really needed someone to care for and about him—that is what friends are for. The boy was hospitalized for several weeks. On his release I saw him coming up the stairs with my son holding the bear. They were both seniors in high school, so this was a very unusual sight!

I asked him what he was doing carrying the bear. He told me that my son told him the story about "Hug Bear" and thought that he needed to borrow "Hug Bear" to help him through his difficult times. Needless to say, "Hug Bear" became an important part of our ongoing family dynamics and the lives of others around us. I said to my colleagues in healing, that I wanted to find a bear that I would bring care, comfort, and healing to my clients and students when the need arises. A bear that I could carry with me to be ready to provide concrete help. That goal and vision haunted me for many years.

Then, Labor Day weekend in 1999, I was on holiday at Myrtle Beach, Virginia. My friend Donna and I were walking through one of the malls on the waterfront late at night and came across a group of people standing in a long line. I said to Donna, "I wonder what all of those people were in line for?" I went over to see and saw that this long line was in a Teddy Bear factory store where adults with a few children at 9:30 p.m. were standing in line to "build" themselves a teddy bear! I said, "There is no way I would ever stand in line to do that."

Curiosity got the best of me and I walked into the store to see what this bear business was all about. The energy captured me and I was hooked! The manager told us that the line was really short that night, as the hurricane scare kept people away. He said that one night the line was so long at closing time (11:00 p.m.) that he told the crowd of people in a line wrapped two times around the outside of his store, that the employees would stay there until the last person had their bears. The shop closed at 3:30 a.m. that night. Now that is what I call a resource for care, comfort, and healing!

I said to Donna, this is where I will find "Hug Bear," and indeed I did. I birthed two "Hug Bears for Healing" that night. The first was HT Hug Bear and the second was EH Hug Bear. I plan to auction the HT Hug Bear at the Healing Touch International meeting January 2000 to raise money for our healing work. Hopefully from year to year we can pass on HT Hug Bear to once again raise money for healing.

The bear that I choose that night is a special edition "Teddy Bear" named after Teddy Roosevelt as Teddy Bears were designed to mark Roosevelt's refusal to kill a bear that had been given to him. The Special Edition Bear marks 100 years of people loving Teddy Bears, I knew that I wanted that energy for my "Hug Bear for Healing!"

2. HUG BEAR MAKES HIS DEBUT

I was teaching EH courses in Gisbon, BC, an island off the coast of Vancouver. The first day's class was "Clearing the Internal Self." I had placed "Hug Bear for Healing" in the center of the circle of the class. When the students questioned me about him I said that I would tell them about him the next day. Little did I know then what was about to happen.

The next day, the class was "Healing Wounds." In the morning meditation (the first thing we do in all of the EH classes to set the stage for the healing and the educational aspect including calling in Divine Source to guide the work) as I was preparing to write guided messages and inspirations to the students, I noticed there was an empty chair in the room. I counted heads to myself and realized indeed everyone was here who was suppose to be there.

I then heard a voice from the bear that said he wanted to participate and be placed in the chair. I promptly got up out of my chair in silence and did just that. Everyone looked at me with curiosity! I went around the room and received a reading for each person. When I got to "Hug Bear" his reading was, "I need someone to hold me!"

The first person who shared their experience was a man from BC. He said that in the meditation he became aware of the only time he was held by his mother was when she cut his hair as a child. Although he knew that she loved him very much, he was never held by her! I invited him to go and pick up "Hug Bear" as HB asked someone to hold him who needed to be held. As the gentleman walked to pick up the bear I remembered that I bought the bear because as mother I was unable to reach my son physically and show him my love. This experience that was recreated out of awareness, helped not only the students healing of not being held by his mother, but also to reaffirm the meaning for me in my own family's healing.

Thus "Hug Bear" made his debut and forever created a place for himself in the EH workshops to give nurturing, caring, and love for anyone who needs it!

3. TRIANGULAR PROCESS WITH HUG BEAR

During the meditation in EH classes in Seattle, WA, I received guidance (similar to what I got before) that Hug Bear wanted to sit in a chair in the circle and be held by someone. This time Shelly asked to hold Hug Bear. I asked for a volunteer to show the class how to assess the Hara Alignment and the Core Star. Many volunteered, but I was led to pick Don, the only male in the group.

Upon describing his issue, Don said he wanted to let go of his ex-wife. He feels he is being held back on his spiritual path regarding unresolved issues with her. In doing the assessment, all of the chakras were open, the energy field was open except the back of the left side and the Core Star was closed. The Soul Seat and the ID point of the Hara were not clear. Both were closed. This data means that emotionally the client is unresolved from past issues. It affects his identity of who he is. In addition, it shows his life purpose is not clear.

I asked his class partner, Shelly, to contribute. She says she knew she was to work with Don as she had unresolved issues with her Dad who never held her. This is the reason she chose to hold Hug Bear.

I then told the class Hug Bear's story. Shelly needed to be held for not receiving parental love. I returned to the client Don and asked if my dialogue with Shelly brought up anything for him. He said that it did. It reminded him about not being able to connect with his children who are on the other side of the country. He said he is not sure they experience his love for them.

I then told another part of my personal story with Hug Bear that was created to send love to my son when he was with his father. I wanted to share my love for him and let him know I was there for him even though I was across the world.

Hug Bear was created to heal my son and me. My son used the original Hug Bear to aid in healing his friend. HB helped our Canadian friend heal from not being held by his mother as related in another story. Today, Hug Bear once again connects the energy of those needing healing from missing out being held and hugged by parents. I have come to understand the importance of hugging between parents and children. If this need is not met, a void can exist that produces pain even years later. Parents, when was the last time you hugged your children?

Mary Jo Bulbrook
Carrboro, North Carolina

Connecting with Jennifer

I arrived home in Newfoundland for the birth of my niece Jennifer. Needless to say, neither she nor her mom were ready for what was about to happen. I was at my parent's home late at night when we got the good news of the baby's arrival weighing in at over 10 lbs. Complications had set in however, as Jennifer was having difficulty being born. The physicians decided that they needed to break her collarbone to be delivered.

I awoke in the middle of the night from a deep sleep with pain in my collarbone. I immediately started working on my collarbone with the intention to send the healing to Jennifer's collarbone. I found out the next day that the doctors were pleased of her progress in healing and that she would have a full recovery. I continued to work on Jennifer each time I saw her and each night as I went to sleep through my own collarbone. Within three weeks her collarbone was healed with no complications.

Donna Duff
Carrboro, North Carolina

The Healing Pillow

One of the things that we teach in Healing Touch classes is the use of energizing something cotton with our hands as love from our hearts to aid in the healing process. Cotton stores energy. I had gotten a cotton-batting pillow for my niece Jennifer who was born with her collarbone broken. I gave the pillow to my brother and asked that they keep it close to Jennifer's collar bone.

Later he told me this story: One night that Jennifer wasn't sleeping well, and crying a lot, my sister-in-law got up several time to try to comfort her, but was unsuccessful. When my brother got up to take his turn walking Jennifer, he noticed that her pillow was not in the crib. Asking his wife where it was, she said in the laundry and it should be dry. My brother got the pillow and put it in her bed. In a short time Jennifer was fast asleep with her comforting "healing pillow."

The pillow was also used for their flight from Newfoundland to Ottawa with Jennifer several months later. Children flying often have trouble with their ears adjusting to the altitude. They often cry in pain on take off and landing. Jennifer had a different experience, as she did not cry at all. The fight attendant remarked to my brother how well Jennifer was doing. So on the way home the pillow was used again with the same results—no crying in pain. My brother called me to tell me the story and wanted to know if the pillow really was the reason that she wasn't crying!

Donna Duff
Carrboro, North Carolina

Newborn Energy

On August 31,1999 our son Cameron Edward was born. After waiting and wondering about him for nine months God gave us a wonderful 7 lb. 2 oz. baby. When Cameron was only one day old our doctor noticed that he was jittery. Tests showed that his glucose levels were low and we would have to increase his feeding schedule to every two and a half hours. He was also a bit jaundiced which caused him to be sleepy. Cameron was just learning to breastfeed and because he was so sleepy, his feeding schedule was very difficult to maintain. We were very worried and decided that some outside intervention would help to give our son some needed energy.

I contacted my sister Donna in North Carolina. She is a Certified

HT Practitioner and Instructor. I was guided by her and an intuitive reading by Mary Jo to administer HT on the right side of the baby's abdomen. To my amazement I could feel the heat coming from that spot. I unruffled it for a few minutes and it cleared. I felt comforted that I could do something concrete to help.

The next day I tried to continue HT, but I felt inadequate and afraid I didn't know enough. So we turned to Cameron's Aunt Liz who practices and teaches Healing Touch therapy. She came to the hospital several times to do healing work. Liz would sweep her hands over Cameron's body, like a gardener would rake a yard. This technique was done to balance the body's energy field. Almost immediately afterwards, Cameron was more willing to eat. Also, his glucose levels rose to normal and he was improving at breastfeeding. His jaundice dissipated after two weeks.

Cameron gained six pounds in two months. We continue to practice Healing Touch on a regular basis to keep his energy field balanced. As with most parents, we worry about our child's health and are willing to do anything that helps maintain good health. It was great to have my sisters as backup and support in caring for Cameron.

Yolanda and Gerard Duff
St. John's, Newfoundland, Canada

Healing the Self

In August of 1999 I was privileged to participate in the Energetic Healing classes IV and V. In EH, I not only learned how to facilitate others in their healing process but I had the delight of working on my own stuff. The classes were taught a week apart thus providing me with adequate integration time for which I was very grateful.

In EH IV (Changing Relationships Energetically) my personal theme for the class was the relationship with myself. As a friend of mine who is a spiritual counselor would say, the relationship between the 10% and the 90% mind. With this class I reviewed my relationship with God. I began a much more intense look at my deepest core issues, knowing that I am not nor have I ever been separated from God, knowing that I am now on a path of surrender. The depth of my self-exploration was not completely revealed to me until the following class (EH V) a week later.

I felt very calm and peaceful after the first class, yet the feeling of incompletion stayed with me for the remainder of the week. In my practice I used what I had learned with some of my clients. While working with them I became aware of many mirrors presented to me through their healing processes. I fully realized that as I "helped" others, I was completing my own work. Yet the missing puzzle piece still eluded me.

The following week I participated in the EH V class (Reshaping Family Energetic Patterns). In the opening meditation I was given a written message which was for each of us in the class.

The Family of One
You are safe.
You are protected.
You are guided in Love.

Be still and know that your Presence
is the Presence of God — each of you.

Each encounter is a sacred reunion.
Each of you is a part of the whole
   — individual, separate —
  yet the whole is within each of you.

Blessings, grace and mercy abound in the
Presence of the Divine,
The Divine within each of you,
The Divine between each of you.

The three of us who were partnering for this work were well matched. Our issues were not identical but were very close. I thought, "Oh, great, here I go again! The same old stuff. Will I never get through this?" I was dealing with long ago childhood issues that I honestly thought I had finished with. I soon realized what I was going to deal with had never even come up.

We began the day by identifying issues linked around our conception and birth. What were our parents lives and relationships like? What types of jobs did they have? Were there other children? On and on the questions came as prompted by the meditation. I was still baffled because I was truly loved and my parents were financially stable. They were healthy, they loved each other and their businesses were secure. The issues that did come up were my mother's previous miscarriage and the fact that forceps had been used during my birth process. It wasn't until the end of the day that I realized just how significant these two issues were.

As my two friends worked with me I felt the energies shifting but no real insights came until the very end. At this time I realized that I felt safe for the very first time in my life and I am 50 years old. I've always felt the need to "protect my back," not really trusting what might be done "to me" when I least expected it. I believe that I had picked up on my parent's apprehension of the possibility of another miscarriage, but then to be literally pulled in such a rough manner from a womb was doubly traumatic. Many things in the early years of my life reinforced these feelings of not being safe. My sister was born when I was 18 months old and my mother had to have surgery six months later. We were sent to live with two aunts in another state during her two month recuperation. By the time I was five, my dad had begun to have blacking out spells. I was neither allowed to ask questions nor was this explained to me. When I was seven he died of a cerebral hemorrhage. Once again nothing was explained.

My healing process began many years ago when in psychotherapy I realized that I thought that my mother had killed my father. As a small child I had heard just enough about my mother having to "terminate life support" for my dad, that it had a tremendous effect on me subconsciously. I thought that I had dealt with this, but until we did the reparenting work, I had no clue that this was still lurking in my system.

It's really interesting that I had already done the forgiveness work and even most of the emotional healing linked with all of this. But it still remained with me energetically and haunted me at all times. It has now been over a month since the class and I feel fantastic. Hindrances linked with my work as an energetic healer and an artist are being addressed with new clarity and focus. My relationship with my family and friends has now shifted as I'm no longer afraid that someone will "leave." My ability to trust has been renewed. My gratitude to Mary Jo knows no bounds for her perseverance and willingness to serve that we might all grow and heal. Thank you, Mary Jo, for this incredible gift that I can now share with so many people on so many levels.

Rebekah Keith
Creedmoor, North Carolina

Brittany

Some years ago when I was quite new to Healing Touch, I was at the home of some friends. Everyone had finished a fine meal, and the children were tired but continuing to enjoy each others company. The adults had settled into an in depth conversation and some fine wine. Out of the corner of my eye I noticed the children playing and wrestling around the lounge. Our hosts eldest daughter Brittany had climbed onto the back of the lounge. Soon after there was a squeal, and I turned just in time to see the little girl do quite a spectacular back flip diving head first into the floor. As expected, her mother was very quick to the scene, but I was puzzled that the qualified health practitioners present were not checking the child. I was prompted to assist with my newly acquired Healing Touch skills. I briefly hesitated, feeling tired and I guess somewhat doubting my ability.

I then asked permission of Brittany and her Mum, and proceeded to do some Unruffling while Mum cradled the child on the lounge. I could see a mark was forming on Brittany's forehead and it began to swell. I was surprised to notice how at ease and accepting the child had become. Everything seemed quiet and peaceful, and I felt encouraged. The little girl soon stopped crying and nestled into her mother's arms. (I'm still amazed how moved I feel recalling this early experience.) After a short period it occurred to me to finish off with some Laser treatment, and soon after the child was taken off to bed.

For the next few days I wondered how Brittany was, but I didn't think to ring. As it turned out I didn't have to. A couple of days later her mother phoned and said how amazed she was at Brittany's recovery. There had been no apparent bruising. The "egg" which was forming on her forehead that night had gone, and even though the mother was convinced there would be a severe concussion, there was very little sign of ongoing discomfort for Brittany.

For me, the lesson was not to doubt, but to trust that the intention of supporting in a situation like this is all one needs.

Craig Pattinson
Beechwood, New South Wales, Australia

My Aunt and Her Headache

"What do you mean you are going to wave your hands around my head?" my aunt said in response to my offer to relieve the pain of her migraine. I was visiting England, the country of my birth, from Australia, paying a visit to my father's sister in a small village in Devon. The pain of her persistent headache was evident on her face, as she battled on to prepare a traditional roast dinner for my welcome home. I had explained a little of the work I was doing, and she had listened politely, though obviously sceptical. (How I like sceptical people! They ask so many leading questions, and are open to new ideas.) I described the principles of Healing Touch in brief and explained that although we cannot see the human energy field, it is just as important to maintain as the parts of ourselves that we can see.

"So, will you let me unruffle your headache and see if you have the standard patterns in your energy field which create migraines?"

"OK. I have nothing to lose, I suppose, as any relief will be a great relief," she reluctantly replied. She sat in her favorite chair next to the slow combustion stove as I gently unruffled and smoothed her tangled aura. Yes, there were several "spikes" so typically present with migraine headaches. We talked of old times and new as she sat quietly, and I continued peeling away the build-up of energy around her head, neck and face areas. "Are you feeling any better?" I asked. "A little," she replied, but not with the excitement I would have expected.

"Well, dear, I have had these bad heads for 30 years now, so I don't expect that waving your hands around will do much. I think I am past helping," she said. I certainly did not agree. I was sure that the HT would provide some relief, and I was sure that my dear aunt was worth helping. The healing herbs and crystals of Aura-Soma finalized my session. The soothing qualities of the violet pomander were gently waved through her aura allowing the energies of color to be absorbed. The next day I phoned to check on my "patient."

"Well, my dear, I slept better than I have for many days, and, yes, my head feels clearer," she reported. "I find it hard to believe that you only waved your hands around me and asked me to take in that wonderful fragrance, and I feel so much better today!"

That was 3 years ago, and aunt has not had another migraine since.

Sue Ashton
Pappinbarra, New South Wales, Australia

Parents Love Us into Heaven

It is a beautiful summer afternoon in July 1998, as I came across the Golden Gate Bridge and traveled into Mill Valley, California where there is an Energetic Healing workshop that I am to attend. Dr. Mary Jo Bulbrook, Founder and Director of the Energetic Healing Program is teaching it.

I am excited about the idea of learning more about the Healing of Mind, Body and Spirit but there is a part of me that is saddened because of my older brother's approaching death. This is resting heavy on my mind. He is suffering from cancer.

I find a congenial group of participants, both women and men, at the workshop, and as we introduce ourselves and share our stories, I mention among other things that my brother has been dying for several months now. Right now the family is struggling how to aid in his transition and there is disagreement how honor him after his passing. This disagreement is causing much pain in me and the family.

I ask if anyone has a cell phone whose number I could give my family in case they need to reach me. Friday passes profitably and without a phone call from my family.

Saturday is a very special day for me. Mary Jo gives the participants a guided meditation followed by a time to continue meditating, while she focuses on each person one at a time and receives a channelled message for each participant. The content we are focusing on for this workshop is "Healing Wounds."

The messages are shared with the group. To my surprise and absolute delight, Mary Jo gives me the following:

Dear Friends,
We are gathered here today to honor you. Let it be known you are important to us, honored and loved for being just who you are.
When you are ready dear child, we will be there to take you to Heaven. Enjoy and know that you are loved.

(Channelled to Sr. Barbara through Dr. Mary Jo Bulbrook, July 18, 1998)

Mary Jo tells me that the message seems not only for my brother regarding his pending transition, but also seems that it is for me too when it is my time to go. She thinks the message is from my deceased father. "Oh, yes," I say. "It sounds just like something my father would do and say." Mary Jo continues to say that I am to give the message to those present when the family gathers for the funeral, if it fits for me to do so.

My brother Joe dies Sunday the very next day after this workshop easing his long lingering illness. It is as if a solution as to how to provide for his transition was needed to bring peace to him and me.

Many years earlier my brother's daughter married into a Lutheran family much to Joe's concern. There were apparently strong feelings between father and daughter about a lot of things. When I read the message at the family gathering from my father given through Mary Jo, I emphasized the first paragraph: "You are honored and loved for being just who you are." Everyone visibly relaxed as they accepted this reading from a Catholic nun to her brother's Lutheran family.

All family members participated fully in the Memorial Mass, there were no issues of Catholic vs. Lutheran. We continued to celebrate life at our Lutheran family's home that afternoon, healing the separation that had started many years earlier.

Sometimes healings happen in unexpected ways. We celebrate and give thanks!

Barbara Cavanaugh, RSM
San Francisco, California

Preparing Nancy for the End of Her Life

Nothing had prepared me for the weeks that I was to spend with my younger sister, Nancy, at the end of her earthly journey. For the last year I had helped her cope with the many challenges she was facing with a dual diagnosis of systemic lupus and cancer. Now she had been diagnosed with inoperable lung cancer with metastasis to her brain and lymphatic system. All of the traditional and complementary medical regimes had been stopped by choice. The essiac, the chemotherapy, the radiation, the prothrombin time—all had come to an end.

"I want you to come and teach me how to die," she pleaded. And so I flew the 1,000+ miles to spend a few weeks at her home. Her request humbled me and my journey was spent in prayerful contemplation that God would guide me in this task. Although sadness at the impending loss pervaded my soul, within my heart there dwelled a sense of honor. At the time of my visit, I had not begun my training in Healing Touch. I was a teacher and practitioner of therapeutic touch, nurse massage therapist and certified Reiki master/teacher, I had a lot of tools, but Nan wanted something different. Although she loved energy work, she wanted real touch.

"Just touch me please. I am so sick of doctors and nurses who are so darn professional. I'm tired of having my body marked with ink," she wailed in an unexpected display of emotion. I was surprised and began to shake. Nan was always the logical, controlled sister, the one from whom I had sought wise counsel. This was not going to be as easy as I thought.

Nothing had prepared me for Nan's debilitated condition. Her hairless head and her shrunken body shocked me. She was unrecognizable. My heart was heavy with pain, my eyes spilled over with tears and we held each other and sobbed. Rocking her in my arms I crooned a favorite lullaby to her calling her my Nanny Goat, an endearing childhood nickname.

Now I had to become objective, put on my professional hat. I quickly assessed that even a light Swedish massage was not indicated. Nan grew to love energy work when she vacationed with me, but now she wanted to be nurtured with actual touch. Together we developed a touching protocol. I now knew that touch and massage were distinctly different protocols. This was her final gift to me. I called it caring touch.

I began by centering and focusing in the present moment. I taught her the relaxation response and used active listening skills. Together we developed a personalized interactive guided imagery with music and color therapy. Most importantly, my touch was administered from the heart. Peace became my demeanor. Calmness pervaded my soul. I focused on total acceptance of Nan's condition as I viewed her as whole and perfect. I consciously had to struggle to let go of my ego and stop trying to fix her. After all, this was my baby sister and her physical presence on this plane was dear to me.

The benefits of touch for Nan were a reduction anxiety and psychosocial isolation that I believe was due to touch deprivation. Her emotional pain and existential loneliness were lessened. We also reestablished a firm loving relationship, one that was always there but had faded with our geographical distance and our years raising children. The most important benefits were an uninterrupted eight hours of sleep and a diminishing of required analgesia. When I arrived she was receiving 200 mg. of morphine p.o. in a 24 hour period. That dosage was gradually reduced to zero until the last days. Nan peacefully made her transition on February 28, 1995, a time that she chose.

Barbara Harris
Osprey, Florida

Changing Beliefs Can Save a Marriage

Tammy is a friend of a friend. She is thirty-something, married with no children and works in an office for a large corporation. I had treated her only once at the friend's house.

Tammy called one evening and asked if I would work with her. She has been experiencing chronic back pain, headaches and TMJ for several years. The doctor just prescribes drugs that have no effect, and at the last visit he suggested breast reduction surgery for the back pain.

At the first session I did "first aid" for the headache, TMJ and backache that was quite helpful, and Tammy felt great when she left. I instructed her to do a pain drain when she feels a headache coming on. She had a good week between the first and second treatments. The shoulder pain was gone and did not come back, the back felt better and there were no headaches.

In the discussion before the second treatment I asked: "How long have you been having the pains?" She replied, "Five years." Then I asked, "What happened five years ago?" Tammy said: "I got married." I thought, "What have I gotten into now!"

In the discussion that followed, two themes evolved. First, Tammy had been active in the performing arts. The pains came on after her old friends called and they discussed their careers on stage and Tammy's career in a corporate office that came with the marriage. Tammy loves the arts, all arts, and the corporate office is not an acceptable substitute. Second, Tammy really wanted children. She felt this was her mission in life. Time was going by, but her job and busy life were too demanding. She knew the time was not now. I suggested she needed to change her belief. We established the following statements:

Old Belief: I am not using all the talents I was given by God.

New Belief: I have faith that all my dreams will be fulfilled.

The session started with grounding vitality to stimulate the field. The key treatment was an energy field drain focused on removing the old the belief and replenishment with the new belief. An inner core balance was used next to stabilize the new belief system. The session finished with a chakra blessing.

I did not see the client again for about two years. She was happy to report no headaches, TMJ or backaches since the last session. She was a new mother with a beautiful baby girl, had quit working for the big corporation and has a part time job working at home as an artist. She is also singing in a local professional choir.

Don Stouffer
Cincinnati, Ohio

Relationship Clearing

This is an interesting divorce story involving the relationship clearing technique, which continually astounds me in it's effectiveness. I had been married for 18 years. My husband, Roger, was a very nice guy and had always supported what I was doing without ever wanting to be involved with it. In 1992 he retired from the Forest Service and took up fly fishing. The same year I started in the Healing Touch program. We gradually grew apart to the point that we had no mutual interests or even mutual friends. Because he never interfered with what I was doing I assumed I was happy, even though I began having lots of dreams about riding bicycles, doing things on my own, and single beds.

I was having lunch one day with a friend from Germany and we were talking about relationships. She said that her last partner of ten years was a very nice guy who adored her but would not participate in any of the spiritual growth things that she was doing. She realized one morning that the thought of spending the rest of her life with someone who wasn't really part of it was appalling to her so she left him. It was like getting hit by a two by four across the head as I realized I felt exactly the same about Roger. I then went to the office and had a Cranio-Sacral treatment. There was a pillar candle of The Virgin of Guadeloupe lit. I thought it was nice, since I have been devoted to Mary for many years. Later that evening I was reading in Andrew Harvey's *Son of Man*. The chapter I had gotten to was the story of the Virgin of Guadeloupe. Too synchronistic! So I meditated and said to Mary, "If you want me to do this you have to make the arrangements." It seems she proceeded to do so. I thought about it for several weeks then had Madeline (a Healing Touch and Energetic Healing practitioner) do a relationship clearing. I asked that Roger understand and accept why I have to do this.

I informed Roger the next Tuesday. He wanted me to give him a chance to get up to speed so when I went to bed that night I was having second thoughts. At 2:00 a.m. I was awakened by a dream of a poster being held up with the words in capital letters "THE END – OVER." No kidding! Then I had a bunch of dreams showing me all the parts of me that I had been ignoring. That evening Roger was telling me the thoughts that he had been stewing about all day. I told him I had changed my mind about giving him another chance. He then looked me in the eye and said, "*I understand and accept why you are doing this.*" These were the exact words from the relationship clearing I had done the week before. It blew me away. The divorce went smoother than my lawyer had ever seen. We didn't fight about anything (we didn't have kids, so that alone made it less complicated). My divorce was final in August and it has been great.

Anonymous

My Sons and Healing Touch

Below is the case study my son Jim did for his HT Level IIA taken in Australia while on tour in 1995 with HT Partnerships. Jim was the only teenager and child with us. His contributions to the group were wonderful as well as the healing he did below! He had taken HT Level I in New Zealand the week before and was taking advantage of traveling with the healing community to learn "officially" HT. Before this time he responded to my healing work like any other teenager. Most of the time he laughed at some of the things I did, but always had respect that it was worthwhile. I was delighted when he decided he wanted to take Healing Touch while on tour. I was even more surprised when he also took Level IIA! See for yourself, how he did.

A is a 39-year nanny who had two cats. She meditates and has seen a HT therapist once a week for the last ten weeks. Her reason for coming today is to learn HT so that she can help others and herself. She has liver problems through blood transfusions, pain in the gut and side, is tired, and has Hepatitis C. Her job is stressful as a nanny. Her partner drinks and does verbal abuse. She just does her own thing. The energy field was eight feet out on the top, left side, bottom and only four feet on the right side. I opened her energy field, connected the chakras and did pain drain over the damaged liver where I felt tingling and throbbing with energy flowing through it. I then Lasered the spot, and gave direct energy. The energy was flowing openly and warm. I also did mind clearing to reduce stress, brushed, grounded and released. In the end all the chakras's were open and very even. The field was even and strong and no problems detected when I hand scanned. — Jim Bulbrook

I am reporting this for several reasons. Not only am I proud at the work he did as a 16 year old, but I want other parents to know teenagers can embrace the work and it will not only help others but change their lives as well. Imagine, a teenager interviewing an older woman and she responded so well! Of course it was a teaching and learning situation, but it was done very professionally. His sensitivity as a beginning practitioner was very good. He was able to actually feel things with his hands and notice when things changed.

The other story I want to share involves my other son Bill who is 23, and currently the business manager of Healing Touch Partnerships. Bill is a graduate in business management from North Carolina State University. He heard of my struggles to find others to help in my business activities as it has experienced tremendous growth. A year ago he announced to me unexpectedly he would like to work for me. I was very surprised and pleased if for nothing else that he would have a good handle on my business as an heir! It has worked out very well for both of us.

A month ago he, his girlfriend Mandy and one of his best friends Eric (who drew the design for Hug Bear for Healing - see related stories), took Healing Touch Level I with Cathy Mack in Carrboro, NC. I have Bill's permission to share with you an e-mail he sent to his friends today. It says something I am very happy to share with you and alert you to about the readiness of young adults for spiritual changes. This was totally unplanned and a wonderful surprise! It represents an important population's perspective on our work that I think we need to address more.

To all: I have shared with all of you about my experiences at Healing Touch Level I. After the experiences that Mandy and I and Eric had, my mom and the other instructors were very interested in the potential impact of HT on young people. We are going to try and plan a special workshop soon focused on our group. Family members and other friends are also welcome.

Recently, I have a whole new outlook on the world and a new found sense of being. If you go into this thing with an open mind, and a sense for greater good, then it will make a difference. You many not take it all for the face value, but that is exactly how it is set up. There is no set thing to take home. You learn certain techniques, but use them in whichever way you are lead. It will affect every one of us differently, but I can assure you that it will do a world of good. Everyone will get their own personal experience and you will take something home with you that you did not have before. This will be part of your journey to lean more about who you are and what it all means.

The other cool thing is that we have arranged a family/student discount rate so the course will be affordable. I want to give it as a gift to you. The changes and awakenings going on in my life right now are unbelievable to me. I know it is related to HT as I believe we are all being guided somewhere, I don't know where yet.

I have just become the Executive Director of the International Alliance for Health and Healing, a non-profit organization dedicated to helping others with their health and healing. I am extremely excited about it. And I just had an absolutely perfect dog come to me that needed someone to care for her and someone to care back. Tonight I sign the adoption papers for her from the Animal Rescue Team. I actually can't say how great I feel things are headed. I want the same great things to happen for all of you. As they are happening for me and this is one small stride in that quest. I feel like Jerry Maguire must have felt after typing that memo in the movie. Some of you may laugh at this, but I want to offer this to you, as I am blessed to have you all as friends, and want the best for each of you. — Bill

A parent couldn't want more for her child—namely, for him to

come into his own spirituality, being very excited about that awareness, directly connecting with God and seeing the influence in his
life, and offering that new awareness to his friends! As a parent, I
believe the best we can do, is to model to our children what is
important to us and then give them our blessings and love to be free
to find their path. Set the energy and they will come.

Jim, Bill & Mary Jo Bulbrook
Carrboro, North Carolina

On the Wings of Angels

It was nearly time. Twenty five years of being a labor and delivery
nurse and I knew Dylan was making a choice to enter the physical
world. His mother embraced each contraction with focus and delib-
erateness. His father watched his mother, marveling at her courage
and strength. They had been here before, but this would be different.
Brianna stayed only three months in their lives, a sweet angel who
came to present herself to her father as his guardian angel and then
return to spirit. But this was different. The genetic studies said
everything was fine.

Dylan eased into our presence and only barely gasped in surprise
at the change in light and sound. *First Rites* by Richard Shulman had
played softly throughout his mother's labor and now his birth.
Someone touched him too vigorously and he cried in dismay. And
then he was held in love and rapture by his mother. Smiling but
silently she stroked him and his father soothed his crown. Dylan
opened his eyes, grasped his father's finger and his mother's breast
and assured them his love would always be present.

That night life changed and Dylan began the same path his sister
had taken. For unknown medical reasons, he too had the same
metabolic disorder his sister had born. But we were not ready to see
that, there must be something else, some other easy issue to treat and
then take him home. Not so, though you see. I began the journey of
preparing him for his return and asking for strength and guidance as
I again helped his grieving parents begin to let go.

Dylan loved the healing light and he brought many healers to his
bedside. To confirm his diagnosis, a liver biopsy was necessary. His
parents did not wish to put him through the painful experience
already resigned that it would be the same diagnosis and outcome.
But the team could not believe it was the same, the tests sent to

Canada and France during her pregnancy could not both be wrong, could they?

Energy healer, Julie Motz, was lecturing in the islands at the time and I asked her if she would consider accompanying little Dylan to surgery. Julie spoke softly to Dylan as they wheeled him from the NICU and apologized to his liver for the insult to its being but reminding the liver that it would be for his highest good to allow the doctor to easily enter his field, his body and remove the wedge. Throughout the entire surgery she provided loving light, holding the intent of healing and apology. Dylan's diagnosis was confirmed, he could not metabolize an amino acid which ultimately leads to deeper and deeper coma and finally death. He spent the next weeks quieting himself in preparation, I assume, for his journey back home.

Janet Mentgen made his acquaintance during grand rounds at our medical center and felt the gap in the Etheric template. He engaged her energy and quietly soothed under her unruffling movements. As Janet repaired the grid, he moved deeper into his relaxed state. Six weeks later Dylan was making physical changes which required his family to make the most painful decision a parent can make. Was it time for more invasive tubes or was it time to let Dylan be with his sister? During the weeks that this special godson of mine was struggling, my beloved Siamese cat was also preparing to leave. I had nursed Ku'u at home with IV fluids for months and one day he looked at me and cried and I knew, no more.

That Sunday we cried together as I held and pet Ku'u. We shared with glee our memories of his many silly antics and spoke of the unconditional love he had given us for so long. Ku'u loved to join in my healing sessions, often resting on the area of the person which was depleted. He was an incredible teacher, my good friend Ku'u. The following day I waited at home for his veterinarian to arrive to help let him go. He laid on my heart chakra all day and we passed that love back and forth between us until it was time for him to leave.

The next day I was present to support Dylan in the same way. I shared with his parents who had made the choice to let Dylan leave, of Ku'u's final day of lesson, giving love without fear. So they held Dylan throughout the day to their heart until the respirator was turned off. The medical staff had prepared them to expect a period of time to elapse while his heart stopped. But no, not Dylan. He left as quietly and easily as he had entered this world. No struggle, no pain, just peace. He took on the mother of pearl colors and in his death glowed. In the NICU room next door where he had spent so many weeks, the parent of another critically ill infant walked over to where I stood outside Dylan's special room. As I cried, she embraced me and asked me to come see Loa, her son.

She shared that moments before she had spent nearly an hour trying to coax him awake. As we walked into the NICU, Loa was looking with wide, bright eyes all around the room. She said she felt Dylan pass through and now the NICU had their own angel. I spoke at my godson's funeral of the many lessons he had taught. But the greatest of all was his lesson of unconditional love. He brought many to his bedside in healing moments. I taught the Chakra Spread to new volunteers and his parents. Each of us was captured by his physical beauty, but more by the beauty of his being. His field was never dense or heavy, only soft and billowing—just as an angel should be, I guess. Fly away little soul, to the light, to the light. Fly away little soul to the light. God is watching, watching. God is watching, fly away little soul to the light.

Lori Protzman
Aiea, Hawaii

Letter to Courtney

Dear Courtney,

I am writing to thank you for helping me become a Certified Healing Touch Practitioner. I used our work together as my case study. When I first met your mother, you were eight years old. I was teaching an introduction to Healing Touch class at the massage school where your mom was learning massage. We were both mothers of special needs children. I was using Healing Touch with my daughter and seeing a new calmness with her. As I told her what I was doing, she invited me to work with you. You sounded pretty sick and I didn't know if I would be able to do anything for you or not.

Your mom impressed me because she knew so much about your condition. She used all the correct medical terms describing your cerebral palsy and medications you were taking. Even though, you were taking the highest doses possible of several medications for seizures, you were still having seizures almost constantly. The doctors had told your mom there wasn't much else they could do for you and you might die soon.

When I started working with you it was difficult for me because it was not like sessions with my other clients. You were so uncomfortable, I couldn't put you on a massage table. I worked while you were in a recliner and I was on the floor. I used chakra connection and modified mind clearing. You moved around a lot and cried. Sometimes your mom would hold you in her lap while I unruffled you. Your mom would say that she felt more relaxed after those sessions.

We met at your house twice a week for many months. You began to have fewer seizures. Then you began to have seizures only when you were sick with a cold or fever. I was able to feel the location in your head where you were having the seizures. I worked to balance this area. You had begun to have more periods where you felt better.

Then one sweet day I visited and heard you laugh. I will never forget that day. You laughed with your whole body and it filled the room with love. I started to cry. That was the day I knew I wasn't just working to help you feel better or to get my certification. I knew you were getting better.

This summer my daughter and I came to your 13th birthday party. You were laughing and aware of all that was going on. Your mom had ponies for everyone to ride. You were able to do what the other kids were doing.

With the help of homeopathy, your mom has you off all your seizure medications. She has taken Healing Touch classes and works on you. You are able to go to school and you use a communication board to help you express yourself. What a wonderful teenager you are becoming.

My heart is filled with love for you and all that you have taught me by letting me share your life. You have taught me to believe not only in the techniques of Healing Touch, but to trust the process. It is for that, I am writing to thank you with all my heart, my sweet Courtney.

Love, Gayla.

Gayla Wood
Chatham, Virginia

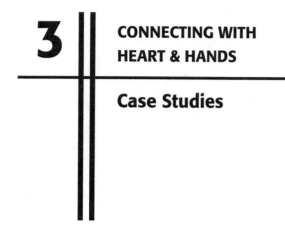

3 CONNECTING WITH HEART & HANDS

Case Studies

Meditation on the Core Star
Bursting forth I reach out to others,
      connecting from the heart.
            Their heart is my heart.

Pulsating beams of light
      dance together the dance of life.
            Waves of joy ripple like the sea.

Expanding outward more and more.
      I am not body.
            I am my higher self.

Sitting in the center,
      quiet calm all around.
            My Star reflecting God's Love for all.

Cathy Mack
Garner, North Carolina

Coping with Breast Cancer

Health care practitioners are some of the worst when it comes to taking care of themselves and I was not one of the exceptions. For several months I put off checking a small breast lump that I felt. I suppose believing that it could not happen to me is the rationale I used to procrastinate getting it checked, but it was more along the lines that I didn't want to take the time out from my demanding schedule to care for the self. The addition of pain and the increase in size convinced me I could no longer deny something was wrong.

The results came back positive and immediate surgery was recommended. The diagnosis was in June of 1995. In a couple of weeks I was scheduled to return to Australia and New Zealand to teach HT. My head was swimming with conflict, input about treatment options, fear in the self and the importance of this diagnosis long term, and fear from my family.

I chose to not tell my colleagues in HT probably out of two reasons: how could an expert in energy work ignore their own health (what would people say), but primarily I didn't think I could cope with many people thinking about me and having opinions what I should and should not do. It was hard enough coping with my families concerns that I could not add anyone or anything else.

I could not think of having surgery right away and I felt that this illness was an attempt to get me off of my path. I had successfully kept HT flowing in Australia and New Zealand with great difficulty on many levels and with personal hardship. The postponement of the trip and courses I was to teach would not only affect this trip, but all of the planning that was in process including a tour of Americans and Canadians to Australia and New Zealand in October/November 1995. It was like a domino effect that moving one piece and the whole system would fall down.

Since I was so indecisive and overwhelmed, I decided to do what I wanted to do and that was complete the trip if I could physically and emotionally, and then have the surgery when I returned in August. I made a promise to my family I would return early if I felt the need to, which is exactly what happened. The last classes in New Zealand were small and I decided to return home several days early.

My surgery was scheduled for August and went smoothly having been prepared pre- and post-surgery by my family and friends. My surgeon was also a friend who knew about HT and his wife was a

Healing Touch practitioner. I asked my surgeon after he operated if he would seal the wound with his hands. He informed me that he always closed his surgery with holding his hands over the wound and turning the healing over to God!

Post treatment options were presented to me including medication and chemotherapy. I told the surgeon I would think about it and give him my answer. Riding home I meditated about my options. When I thought of the chemotherapy I immediately visualized a fist smashing me in the face and knocking me over. When I thought of the medication I saw me swimming with cement blocks on my feet! During the week I thought about it again and came up with similar reactions. So I decided to not take any other treatment.

The most significant experience related to this story takes place several years before any symptoms. I had sponsored the HT support group in my office. One night I was being worked on by one of my friends at the end of the evening. She was doing Magnetic Unruffling and was not able to get my energy clear over the breast area. She told me this as she kept struggling to get it clear. It was near the end of the study group time so I said, "It doesn't matter, we don't have time." She worked a little while longer without much success.

Several days later I had thoughts about a relationship issue that was conflicted. I had not thought of it in many years. I was puzzled why I was thinking of this issue until I remembered the experience of receiving Magnetic Unruffling and not being able to get clear! It showed me the power of energy work to pick up energy blocks before they manifest themselves in the physical. Even with this insight and the fact of being a psychotherapist I did not then take steps to do anything else about this conflict!

When I received the diagnosis of breast cancer I took time to think about what may be related to the root of this problem. I once again thought of the same conflicted relationship! To me this clearly established the link of energy work, problems in the emotional body and disease process!

Six month later the woman who worked on me returned to North Carolina for the holiday and called me. While chatting I said that I didn't think she had heard about my bout coping with breast cancer. She gasped and became very agitated saying how sorry that she was that she did not clear me doing Magnetic Unruffling during our support group. I laughed and said that she tried and did exactly what a practitioner needs to do—give the client information, suggest what needs to be done. I did not do anything with the information I received that I was not clear energetically. A practitioner is only expected to do their best. This seemed to calm my friend.

Later on in the conversation she reported that summer she had trouble with her breast hurting but the tests did not show anything. I laughed again and said that because she had not separated clearly from me she picked up my symptoms. Important lessons for us both! Although the surgery went smoothly and I healed rapidly, I was not prepared for the numbness throughout the entire arm and subsequent loss of feeling and nerve sensation. I am sure I must have been told about this but I know the implications did not sink in until I actually experienced it.

Ten days post surgery I was back teaching HT IIIA in Durham, NC. Someone from the group introduced me to trying crystals to absorb the congestion in the arm and see if it would affect the numbness. I have never used crystals for healing. As a health care professional this seem to stretch a point for me. I enjoyed having crystals around, but would not consider using them for healing.

After holding the crystal on the arm for several hours as I was sitting in class teaching, I was astounded that the place where the crystal was there was no longer any numbness but tingling. I decided that if it can clear one spot, it can clear the whole arm! I continued to use it on the arm and eventually all the numbness was gone and nerve sensitivity not only returned to the arm but to the chest wall as well—something I was told would not happen.

From my personal experience I can say there is definitely a benefit that is not mere coincidence! I really don't think I would believe it if I had not experienced it then and later.

Mary Jo Bulbrook
Carrboro, North Carolina

Lessons and Insights:
Having breast cancer has taught me a lot that I want to pass on. I will list the learnings in the form of principles and suggestions:
1) Physical illness can show up in the energy field before manifesting physically.
2) There is a link between emotions and physical illness.
3) Unresolved emotions will manifest as congestion, thick and sticky in the field.

4) Magnetic Unruffling from HT and Energy Field Drain and Replenishment from Energetic Healing are two treatments of choice to removing blocked energy. Ultrasound, Therapeutic Touch, and Unruffling are also effective. This works for blocked energy from emotions and physical causes such as anesthesia and medication.
5) Energy work speeds healing.
6) Energy work decreases the need for pain medication.
7) Surgery creates a tear in the energy field that needs to be repaired by sealing the wound.
8) Over the surgical site the etheric layer needs to be built up by slowly placing the hand over the area at the etheric level and rebuilding the damaged etheric mass.
9) The chakras at or near the surgical site needs to be cleared and repaired.
10) The Hara Alignment usually needs to be healed.
11) The meridians that travel through the surgical site needs to be repaired and cleared.
12) Crystals can clear congestion and facilitate the return of nerve damage.

My Teacher as Healer

I have always admired SR my high school teacher and a special friend. SR was a Catholic Nun who I was very close to in my young adult life. I heard that she had developed a rare case of leukemia and was not able to continue to teach which she loved to do. I was now not living in the same town as SR and only got to visit her on my trips home. On one of those occasions, I was told by the Sisters that SR was not doing very well and having a lot of pain. They said she was not seeing visitors but she would see me. I was very honored to have been able to visit with SR this trip.

I remembered the good old days we had together. I had help her with doing the high school year book. SR was a great photographer and took all the pictures during the school year. In the summer we put it together by ourselves. We had a lot of fun doing the yearbook and sharing good quality time together.

Her room was in a beautiful setting in the convent, with lots of soft colors and flowers. As I entered her room I could feel the sense of loneliness. Her pain was very high. She was experiencing pain in all her joints and back. I greeted her with an eagerness do some Healing Touch to help relieve her pain. I worked with her for about an hour but was not sure how she was experiencing the treatment. She gave little feedback and I could see she needed to sleep. I asked if it was OK to return tomorrow to visit. "That would be nice," she said.

That night, I prayer to God for a healing to help her rest and free her of pain. I arrived the next day for our visit and SR was sitting in a chair petting her brother's dogs that she loved. I was so happy to see she was feeling better. When her brother left she said the pain was still there and she doesn't like to let the family know how much pain she is in. So I offered another healing session and she was a little more open to receive. I was able to help some, but not enough for all the pain to leave.

I once again prayed for healing and guidance to do the best techniques for pain. I got to return the next day to see SR and once again I did a healing session on her. This time she said that she was glad I was there to visit with her but wasn't sure how much it really help the pain. It was time for me to leave SR that night and I wasn't sure if I would see her again because I was returning to NC in a few days.

I was now feeling a sense off discouragement that I didn't help SR's level of pain. I felt I should have been able to relieve the pain with all the healing techniques I know. I thought this healing doesn't always work! And where was God?

The next day I got a call from one of the Sisters to thank me for being with SR. Sister said for the first time in months SR felt well enough to join them for community prayer and that her level of anger was much less these past few days. I was speechless and overwhelmed!

Once again SR taught me great lessons: 1) To get out of my ego and not be attached to the outcome. 2) To know our prayers are always answered maybe not the way we want them to be. 3) Our teachers and mentors will always be there to teach us the important lessons.

This experience and has truly made me a better healer. To know that all healing is not physical, we need to remember the emotional, mental, and Spiritual. To SR, my gifted teacher as healer, I hope and pray she still will watch over me as a guarding angel and continue to teach me from the other side.

Donna Duff
Carrboro, North Carolina

An Interesting Twist

A woman I had known at work called and asked if I would see her son who has Tourette's syndrome. She had heard that Healing Touch might help calm him and help control his movements. I treated him several times, was pleased to see him improve, but suggested he receive cranial sacral treatments to further stabilize his nervous system. She followed this suggestion and he experienced significant relief.

Meanwhile, the boy's father was so impressed with his son's improvement that he called to ask if I would see him for his acid reflux condition. He had been medicating under a physicians care for over a year, but had not seen any improvement. He was otherwise very healthy and couldn't understand why he had this problem. Our first energetic assessment indicated that his second and third chakras were compromised in the front and closed in the back and his Hara line looked like a large S. His field was dense and congested over his chest, throat and legs and several energy blocks were found near the esophagus. It took considerable work to balance his system! For the first treatment we opened his system with a spiral meditation, cleared his field with Magnetic Unruffling, opened his chakras with a chakra connection, balanced the core chakras and straightened the Hara line with the basic balance (Cath Webber-Martin) and used Ultrasound to aid healing of the throat and esophagus. He felt "lighter" around the chest and had much more energy than when he arrived. He thought this treatment might work!

During his second visit we taught him the Hara meditation to help keep his chakras open and his stress level down. The inflammation in his throat and esophagus seemed to have diminished energetically. He confirmed that he had felt so much better after his first Healing Touch treatment that he thought he would like to learn this himself. We gave him a schedule of classes and both he and his wife registered and took HT Level I in the next available class. They use their knowledge mostly to help their two sons.

At his next visit he revealed his job caused him a lot of stress and he never really relaxed even at home. We decided an Energy Field Drain and Replenishment might help. After explaining it, he agreed to try. We asked him to think about the causes of his stress at work while we drained the energy from his feet. When the field cleared he felt like he had "let go" of some of this baggage. We replaced his anxiety with the suggestion that he "be still" and know that God is with him and he can trust in Him. His wife called two days later to say that he had called her at work to tell her people were smiling at him at his office. "I can't believe he even noticed it," she said! Several days later she called again to say that while they were taking a walk after dinner he commented on the beautiful sunset. In their 16 years of marriage she had never heard him say anything so esoteric. What were we doing to him?

When he returned for his next visit, he said our treatments had really helped him put his work environment in perspective. Did we think we could help him with his son? He felt the boy was always trying to cross him, violating the house rules, and their exchanges were loud, angry and very unsatisfying. We agreed to try another Energy Field Drain and Replenishment. This time he had many emotional experiences that led him through an intensive examination of his attitude toward his son, his inability to cope with his demands and his unwillingness to relax his control. He suggested we replace his stress with love and understanding. He began to see his relationship, as a father to his son, could be different. It was a life changing experience. A year later he and his teenage son are "friends" who can discuss events and activities without ugly exchanges and actually enjoy each other's company.

He still, however, experiences the acid reflux from time to time, but he has been off medication since his first Healing Touch treatment. His physician has told him to continue the energy work as it was doing more for him than any medical treatment he could give. He is continuing to work on his belief system and letting go of detrimental life experiences one at a time. He continues to grow!

Joan C. Stouffer
Cincinnati, Ohio

Energy Healing in the Surgical Suite
    When I first saw Kaye she was very anxious and tense. For two months she had felt like she had a lump in her throat when she swallowed or coughed and had been to her internist and ENT specialist for diagnoses. She was told she had a swollen larynx or maybe gastric reflux. The special diet she was given did not help. After two months an X-ray was taken and the new diagnosis was a

tumor on her esophagus. At this time she was so anxious she couldn't sleep and was seeking ways to relax.

My assessment indicated a collapsed and compromised energy field with chakras 5, 6 and 7 closed. The energy at the throat felt like a pencil with the point at the front of the neck not at all like a tumor. A Full Body Connection reenergized her chakras and field; Ultrasound, and clearing and balancing the throat chakra relaxed the throat muscles and integrated previous scars from herniated ruptured disc surgery ten years previous. The client felt much calmer and was able to swallow better, but a "feeling" remained.

During the subsequent six weeks of Energetic Healing and Healing Touch, Kaye was able to sleep comfortably and eat well, but knew the "tumor" was still there. Further testing, including an EKG, by her physicians hypothesized the tumor was a fluid filled sac that could be drained. However, an MRI and sonogram failed to find it. Each time I assessed her with my hand I continued to feel the pencil so we knew something was there. A CAT scan finally indicated a bone spur emanating from the spine at the C-7 vertebra and protruding into the esophagus. Surgery was scheduled to remove the spur.

When the client requested Healing Touch in recovery, the physician suggested the practitioner be invited into the surgery suite during the procedure. I excitedly accepted the invitation. In the pre-op area we strengthened her core energy with an Inner Core Balance and talked to her body to prepare it for the trauma of surgery. She was quite relaxed as we entered the surgical suite with the physician. When the physician showed me the pictures of the bone spur, I was amazed to see it looked just like the pencil I had felt energetically at my initial assessment.

While the team prepared Kaye for surgery, I held her feet and sent energy through her body keeping the system energetically stimulated and "silently" talked to her heart, lungs, skin, nervous system and blood explaining to each what to expect and how I wanted them to react. When the surgery began I moved to about 12 inches above her head and held her energy field throughout the procedure. I continued to silently talk to her, encouraging her to remain calm. As the procedure started her blood pressure was about ten points lower than the physician ordered, so again I silently asked her heart and blood to increase the pressure as needed. The pressure rose and remained steady throughout the surgery. When the final stitches were in place, the anesthetist said, "OK, tell her she can wake up now." I placed my right hand on her head and silently told her the surgery was over and she could wake up. Well! She did! The breathing tube and monitor leads were still in place, which caused the nursing team to scramble. As soon as the tube was removed Kaye said, "I want to see Joan. Come over here." She was fully awake! I held her hand while final preparations for removal to the recovery room continued.

In recovery I cleared her field of the remaining anesthetic with Magnetic Unruffling, relieved the small amount of pain at her throat with a Pain Drain and used Ultrasound to heal and integrate the scar. Kaye had no nausea or discomfort and was mentally alert. There was no bleeding or oozing at the scar. When she was taken to her room, Kaye got out of bed to use the toilet with no repercussions except the nurse's dismay. She slept well through the night with no medication and was discharged in the morning after eating a full breakfast. She returned to her responsibilities at home. I saw her in seven days for follow-up. The scar was only visible if examined closely and she felt great. There was still some "feeling" in her throat that seemed to be sensation from the trauma of the surgery. She had no problem eating or speaking, but couldn't sing high notes yet. Energetically, her field was free of the pencil point. I used Ultrasound to reduce any swelling that may have remained internally and an Energy Field Drain and Replenishment to address the fifth chakra issues that could be causing the recurring medical conditions. She felt that her inability to speak up and express her feelings could be the cause. She was relieved to finally be addressing it.

Joan C. Stouffer
Cincinnati, Ohio

My Aching Back
Jimmy is a 37 year old father of two. He had been in an automobile accident three years before I saw him for the first time. He had been thrown out of his van when the seat belt broke and landed on his left side in a ditch along the road. His T-7 vertebra was broken, but the spinal cord was uninjured. His lower back, knees and ankles were not noticeably injured, but are now stiff in the morning or after periods of inactivity.

He travels on airplanes frequently for work and loves to play golf. Both of the activities were causing him so much discomfort that he was rarely playing golf. He had to travel. Physicians had treated him with medications for pain and muscle relaxation and a chiropractor had given spinal adjustment. He achieved some temporary relief, but not as much as he wanted. He believed he should be pain free.

Energetically I found his field to be full of congestion around his back and shoulders, the spine closed and hip, knee and ankle chakras compromised. For his first experience with Healing Touch I cleared his field with Magnetic Unruffling, opened the leg chakras with a chakra connection and relaxed the back muscles with a vertebral spiral. Finding a sharp spike at the lower back, I then used the Hopi Technique to repair the damage evident there. From that first treatment Jimmy had increased flexibility in his neck and shoulders and his lower back felt really good. He committed to a return visit.

At the second visit I repeated the treatments as the pain had returned in his back, but talked to him more about the accident. He became emotionally upset when talking about it arousing my suspicions about the impact of the accident on him in mind and spirit, not just body. A friend and I told him about the Full Body Connection with autogenic response and asked if he would be willing to try this treatment. He agreed.

At a third session we discussed the accident in detail and led him through it while exercising the full body connection. He became very relaxed, had several energetic releases at known pain sites and fell asleep, but he did not release emotionally. I felt he needed some time after this treatment to think about the accident and integrate this work.

A week later he called and asked if I would see him again. This time I suggested he think about his mental attitude about the accident then and now. He revealed that he was still angry with the person who had hit him because there was never an apology from the driver who was clearly at fault and had caused him such pain. I explained to him how a treatment called an Energy Field Drain and Replenishment might help him release this anger and replace it with inner peace. He was ready. As he thought about the accident and the driver, I began to drain the stress from his field through his feet. He felt energy leaving his body in "waves," became very emotional and began to cry. I felt large chunks of energy fly from his body. I cleared the field three times before the energy was stable. He could no longer think of the driver or the accident. We replaced the anger with peace in understanding that the driver may have been too embarrassed or stressed to apologize and that the problem remained with the driver not Jimmy. He was exhausted but felt more like himself than he had for three years.

I saw Jimmy three weeks later at church. He was happy to tell me that he had no back pain even though he had taken three trips on airplanes since I had treated him and he was playing golf several times a week. The stiffness in his legs had disappeared too. He was surprised that his mental attitude about the accident and the driver had such a profound effect on his physical being. It was a convincing experience for me too. Energy work is powerful and demonstrates the connection between mind and body.

Joan C. Stouffer
Cincinnati, Ohio

Chris's Transformation

As a pediatric physical therapist in a public school setting I encounter many challenging situations while caring for children with multiple disabilities. I use a combination of traditional PT and energetic interventions in order to help my students progress to their optimal potential. The following experience with Chris is one I will not forget for a long time.

Chris arrived at school in great distress. He was slumped forward in his wheelchair. His eyes were closed and he was minimally responsive. Because Chris is non-verbal, we were unable to ask him what was wrong. However, after getting him out of his wheelchair, we knew exactly what was wrong. Chris's face was dirty, his clothes were urine stained and he had feces smeared on his trunk and legs. I was scheduled to have Chris for physical therapy at that time but I knew he needed to be cleaned more than what the assigned task was. His teacher asked if I would give him a bath during our session. Without hesitation I agreed. No one should have to experience the discomfort and humiliation of that situation. After the bath and hair wash, Chris looked better physically. However, he still wasn't smiling. He was sitting with his head to his chest and appeared very depressed.

I had less than five minutes left out of a thirty minute session. I knew a physical therapy intervention wasn't going to improve Chris's day. I thought, however, an energetic intervention might. So I set Chris on his back on a mat, and gently gave him a Chakra Blessing which is part of the Energetic Healing program whose goal is to bless and heal. With each pass over his body, I spoke his name and offered a blessing or encouragement. When the technique was finished, I picked Chris up and held him on my lap. I whispered, "Chris, you are a child of God. You are good. You are smart. You are strong." With that, I gave him a squeeze and positioned him in his wheelchair. Chris smiled sat erect and held his head high. He was changed and from that day on, and I too am changed. Now I knew how important energy work is, in helping one feel better about themselves!

Jean Gustafson
Scotia, New York

Lessons and Insights:
1) Meeting physical needs are primary before one can go to higher level needs.
2) Those with disabilities have feelings that need to be met. People often override these because of the overwhelming demand for physical care.
3) Energy work can dramatically change how we feel about ourselves.
4) Take time to bless the self and others.
5) A lot can be done in 5 minutes to change one's whole perspective.

Altering the Experience of Cystic Fibrosis

Bart is a 24 year old man with the congenital disease Cystic Fibrosis (CF) which is a life threatening, terminal, and very debilitating disease. Bart's mother asked me to see him in my private nursing practice to balance the effects of the disease and medical treatments. Although Bart has struggled his entire life, he is an actor and author involved in creative writing for children. However he now is unable to work and is on a disability pension. HT started on October 9, 1998 and is ongoing covering two sessions prior to a lung transplant and three in the first postoperative week. Bart is on a large number of drugs to fight infection and enhance respiratory function. His deepest stresses were physical and his little-expressed fear of the lung transplant and death. Bart has difficulty resting due to respiratory problems and pyrexia. Bart used to meditate and work with chakras which "felt good," but now he has no energy and cannot concentrate. He is highly responsive to energetic work.

A hand scan assessment revealed energy was collected around Bart's head to about 12 inches, and protruding from his back over the shoulder blades. It felt full and congested. "Sticky" energy was felt over his lungs both front and back. On reassessment I sensed the front lung area was full of a gray fluffy substance. The Solar Plexus area felt empty and there was an area of heat over his left thigh. Over all energetic state was of great depletion especially in the lower half of the body where it was very find and barely one inch from his body. All the chakras from the heart down especially the root and feet were very weak and compromised. He was very ungrounded.

I used Therapeutic Touch, (to clear the congestion around his head and back), Unruffling and modulation, Magnetic Unruffling, (for greater depth of cleansing especially over the lungs that was resistant to moving and to clear the medications and their effect on the energy field) Laser and Ultrasound (to break up congestion). I energized the foot chakras to increase grounding and to help then open and strengthen. I was guided to cleanses and energize Bart's heart chakra. Bart asked what he could do to ground and increase his energy. I guided Bart to visualize himself as a tree with his feet or roots going deep into the soil to ground and bring up earth energy and his arms and head as branches taking in the sun. (This connected into Bart's strong sense of the sun as a source of energy.) I suggested that Bart learn to trust that energy will flow if asked, that no effort is needed, and the value of trusting in his own inner knowing, of "letting go" and resting in that knowing. At the end of the session Bart had a coughing fit which disrupted his very peaceful state. Therapeutic Touch was used to calm and soothe that field so he settled quickly. Overall he felt much better in the chest, more relaxed and less tight with pain in the shoulders and leg removed. He felt the session had been of benefit and wanted to continue.

Two more session were done in the hospital. Over all he felt more balanced and relaxed for a few hours after HT. Some benefit lasted for about 24 hours, as Bart felt less scattered in this time. He was also more energetic. On a well being scale of 0 to 10 he usually changed from 3 to 5. Our goals were to continue to strength the energy system. He increased his activity and this overtired him. It was clear he needed more treatment regularly and would benefit from increased sessions. Therefore I taught his carer to do energy work with him.

After his 12th session, Bart was scheduled for a lung transplant that took seven hours. He was exhausted and whispering, and had a great difficulty swallowing and coughing. There was a wound from armpit to armpit along the breast line, four chest drains and his pain was not well controlled. He had huge does of immunosuppressive drugs. The energy was very full with a great sense of pressure that pushed out against my hand nearly two feet especially around the chest area. There were holes found over the wound and drain sites. Most of the chakras were either closed or compromised. The throat was full of pressure and out to 1.5 feet while the others were depleted. However the sacral and root were still stronger than before surgery. It is as if his will to live was strengthened, as was his emotional more stabilized. After treatment Bart felt more relaxed, the pain was considerable reduced, and coughing was improved. The blood pressure also has improved. The energy smoothed and the chest area filled very easily. The chakras all opened more vigorous but were counter clockwise. This seems good as they were in balance being all the same size and speed. He progressed well with energy work working hand in hand with his regular medical regimen. Over time the benefits became obvious and the impact of energy work was evident.

Initially Bart's energy system was incredibly depleted and fragile. He was in major physical breakdown and great fear. The major benefit he gained was a reduction of the physical symptoms, relaxation and pain relief. When he was very physically compromised these benefits lasted for a short period of time. On reflection, daily HT work was needed in conjunction with medical therapies, to combat the effects of the persistent infection. Despite this he was able to move forward emotionally to verbalize his fear of dying and to face a lung transplant and possible death calmly. Post operatively, Bart's progress was excellent especially considering the magnitude of the surgery and his very poor physical state. HT appeared valuable in balancing the effects of his major problems, many being iatrogenic. His wound healed quickly and he was discharged in less than three weeks. His voice improved.

Physically his body has changed, his shoulders have opened up and legs are stronger. Bart feels that HT has been of considerable benefit and a significant factor in his progress. HT enhanced his ability to cope and supported his own inner strength. He stated "I am a strong person, used to a lot of pain." He reported he had been preparing his body for the transplant for a long time and said, "Then you came along." I intuited that he meant just when he needed the additional support. On refection I felt that Bart's goals were met. HT helped him considerably at a physical, emotional and a spiritual level. He feels he has grown and strengthened as a person, he said recently "I know who I am not. Our goal of enhancing the healing process was certainly achieved and changed the course of his illness!

Jane Hall
Melbourne, Victoria, Australia

Caring for Dad

My dad, at 77 years of age, was scheduled for quadruple bypass surgery for cardiac arterial blockages. Two years prior Mom had passed about a week shy of their 53rd anniversary, and now he lived alone with his cat. I lived nearby. I offered Healing Touch when I found out about the surgery. Dad is an extremely intelligent individual with a degree in biochemistry, three years of medical school, and over 50 years as a business entrepreneur, so I was a little surprised when he agreed on a series of pre and post heart surgery treatments. He said that he couldn't understand how Healing Touch works, but that, "It couldn't do any harm!"

At our first session, his breathing was slightly labored and his skin was pasty. Our short term goals were to stimulate relaxation, ease pre-surgical nerves, and reduce post-op pain. My goal was to help create a healing environment for the surgery, Dad, and the surgical team, as well as giving a daughter's love and support.

I had planned to do a Chakra Spread because of the transforming nature of the surgery, however, I intuited the instruction "not yet." Assessment showed a field close to the body with increased flattening of the field around the throat, heart, and solar plexus. The chakras were energetically unbalanced with blockages in throat and root. I felt a strong prickly sensation between the left atrium and right ventricle, and sensed energy moving slowly, with low vitality. I have come to interpret prickles to indicate congestion, and pins and needles, or spikes, to indicate pain or discomfort.

Because of a move up in surgery, the first session was done as a distance healing in an isolated corner of a private waiting room. During the procedure, I sensed fear and resistance from both Dad and the heart organ. Following the Chakra Connection and modulation to the heart, I sent love and gratitude, and a prayer for fulfillment of the highest good as part of my goal of supporting a healing environment. Then I turned my attention to the OR environment. I connected heart-to-heart with the surgeon and anesthesiologist, and envisioned their fields filling with light and love. I sensed a great cohesive heart energy coming from the surgeon as he approached the side of Dad's body. Then I saw a vision of a flash of light beams emanating from below the feet through the crown of each member of the surgical team. The fields between Dad and the entire surgical team intermingled, creating a very large blended field of light. As my heart expanded, I withdrew my connection from the group, re-centered, and ended the distance healing, knowing that Dad was in the best of hands.

Following the 4 1/2 hour surgery, Dad's surgeon reported extensive arterial blockage, necessitating a quintuple bypass. However, he said he was pleased with how smoothly the surgery went. Dad was doing fine, his vital sings were excellent, and the veins used for the bypass held up very well.

I went to the ICU for session #2 for Dad. He was unconscious and on a respirator. His skin was pale, but his breathing was regular. The field was distorted in shape and vitality. It was full and strong in the upper body, and shallow and weak below the sacral. There was a feeling of warmth over the heart, but the rhythm was even and strong, unlike the pins and needles disturbance and low vitality assessed before surgery. There were pins and needles over the sternum, and a feeling of static over the lower abdomen. There was a blank, or empty, energy pocket with prickles down the right leg, close to the knee and above the ankle. I later found out that the saphenous vein had been removed to be used as the bypass. For the treatment session I used Magnetic Unruffling to clear the field. Then, I used Ultrasound over the areas of incision for wound sealing, as well as working on congested energy in the legs, until I felt the energy disturbance break up and smooth out. I did a few other techniques, and as his field filled with energy, Dad's arms and legs jerked, and he opened his eyes. His color returned to his face and body.

The nurse reported that his vitals were improving rapidly from the moment he opened his eyes and came out of the anesthesia. As a result, the respiratory doctor discontinued the respirator ahead of expectations. Dad's only complaint was some heaviness in his left shoulder. He said he had no pain. He was scheduled to be in the ICU until the next morning, however the cardiac team doctor cleared him to be moved to the cardiac ward about 5 1/2 hours after the quintuple bypass surgery. When I left him that night, Dad was alert, seemed relaxed, and continued to be pain free.

The next session was again in the hospital. Dad said he had no pain. He had requested a sleeping pill to block out hospital noise so he could get some sleep. He was coughing and clearing his lungs with very little problem. He was alert, with good coloring, but looked tired, and the tone of his voice and facial expression showed frustration. He explained that with having some abdominal gas buildup, and wanting to have the last catheter removed. The goal for the day's treatment was to reduce stress, speed healing, return to normal his digestion and excretory function, and to increase vitality. I implemented this with Chelation.

During the day the remaining IV and catheter were discontinued. The gas pain was gone. Dad had walked a lot, and was still pain free. His nurse told us that as a result of such rapid progress, he was being moved to a transition suite. It was thought provoking to find out that two other bypass patients of Dad's surgeon were in the same cardiac ward, were younger than Dad, experienced a lesser surgery, but were not faring nearly as well. Both the other patients were in pain, on pain medication, and only minimally ambulatory.

We were both shocked the next morning when Dad was discharged after only three days. He was scheduled to receive two weeks of home nursing, however Dad never needed this care because of his rapid return to normal vital signs. His appetite had been healthy from the day following surgery, and his surgeon commented that for his age and complexity of surgery, he had resumed normal activities at an extremely rapid pace.

Over the next six months, dad had his medications reduced, and rarely felt the kind of depression over Mom's loss that had prompted him to use anxiety medication. Plus, he is now walking about three miles five days per week, eating healthy, and we are able to share together special times. I am always so awed by the power and love in energy work, and I am so grateful.

Barbara Rulf
Springfield, Virginia

Fibromyalgia: A Quick Fix Story

Judy was referred to me by another of my clients She was 53 years old, but had one of those plump, ageless faces that belied her chronological age, despite the severe pain and disability she was suffering. She entered my office barely able to move the walker that supported her. She had great difficulty getting onto and lying down on my well-padded massage table. She had a long history of medical problems that seemed to have begun with an attack on her by some students at the high school where she works, several years earlier. She ended up being trapped in an elevator with a heavy dose of Mace sprayed at her. Since then, she had severe allergies and asthma, requiring use of heavy doses of steroids, respiratory inhalers, anti-anxiety drugs and now pain-killers. She then developed diabetes in response to the heavy prednisone levels.

Her energy field felt like it was surrounded with barbed wire and broken glass. As I worked to Unruffle this sharp edge, the client wept silently. I worked on her for about 45 minutes, explaining at the end that she might continue to have emotional releases, physical detox reactions, and that she should be aware that sometimes medication dosages may need to be adjusted as a client begins to heal. I encouraged her to call me if she had any questions or problems before her appointment the following week. I heard no more. The next week, an apparently totally different person arrived for her appointment. If I hadn't had her name on the schedule, I wouldn't have known her. She moved freely without a walker, her color was rosy, and she was smiling and chatty. She had quite a week in the interim. She went home, feeling extremely tired after the treatment. She slept for four hours, and awoke feeling refreshed and wonderful. She felt so good, she decided to wash the windows while she could move. Then she developed chest pains and feared she was having a heart attack. She called 911 and was taken to the hospital. All the tests proved negative for a coronary, but they decided she was grossly overmedicated, and cut back on all her medications. They observed her overnight and sent her home the next day.

She proceeded to develop flu-like symptoms, but this time she recalled my warning and began to pay attention to what these symptoms might represent in relation to her personal and emotional life. She recognized she had a lot of unresolved resentment in her marriage, and grief. She called her therapist, whom she hadn't seen in several years and arranged an appointment. During the week at work she recognized how she had taken everyone else's responsibilities. She began giving back those jobs that were not hers. She made amends with her son over a situation in which she had unfairly accused him of something. She identified areas of her marriage that needed attention. As she shed these long-held burdens, her pain subsided. She ate more fresh vegetables and less junk food. She was still aware of some residual pain, but it did not incapacitate her as it had for the previous three years.

I recommended she continue weekly treatments for one month, and then go to monthly for several months. In the meantime, I would teach a friend or family member to do some energy treatments to support her between visits. Judy came in for two more treatments, and then stopped. I learned from her friend that she was not able to sustain the progress she had made, and gradually over the next year, went back to her old patterns of doing too much, eating too much, and the pain returned. She did not seem able to ask for help again. My lesson was to remember that I am simply a facilitator. I can lead 'em to water, but I can't make 'em drink. I take comfort in knowing that she found the way once, and perhaps she will want to find her way back at some time in the future.

Mary Ellis
Olympia, Washington

Affecting Arthritis

Talon is a part Native American nurse who experienced great pain in both knees from arthritis. He had volunteered to be the demo for the class while I was demonstrating Pain Drain. The next day while talking with the coordinator of the Healing Touch class about other things, he shared that he had been pain free for 24 hours and did not require medication, something very unusual for him. His wife was so surprised that she is willing for him to take more HT classes and even wants him to work on her mother!

Bernie Clarke
Olympia, WA

Lessons and Insights:
1) Demonstration of effectiveness of HT is what wins people over including not only the client but family and friends as well. This is an example of why HT and EH has grown so quickly and so rapidly even reaching out to the non-believers.
2) Chronic illness can be influenced with even dramatic changes in a very short time. In other instances, however, chronic illness needs repeated treatments on a regular basis.

What's Easter Without Lilies?

Diane, 35, is an old friend that was spending Easter day and evening with us in Cincinnati. She has taken Healing Touch Level I and we have treated her several times.

After dinner while cleaning up in the kitchen Diane came in contact with an Easter lily, became very light headed and almost passed out. I immediately removed her from the kitchen, sat her down and held the energy to stabilize her field. She responded very well to removing the lily, and we agreed on a treatment later in the evening after the other guests had gone.

The initial assessment later that evening showed that her field was totally closed (pendulum still). The seven chakras, Hara line, Core Star and aura were closed. The aura was very thick and sticky over the chest and head. I started the treatment sequence with Magnetic Unruffling to remove the toxins left in Diane's system from the lily. I could smell the lily on my hands and the thickness in the field changed with Unruffling. The field was clear and fully open when I finished Unruffling. At this time I brought the Easter lily back in to the room and sat it on a chair next to her head. Immediately her eyes began to water, her head became thick with congestion; her breathing became more difficult and a piercing headache developed. I began a Lymphatic Drain since the allergic reaction to the lily is an immune system dysfunction. Since most of the reaction was in the head and upper torso I did most of the work in this region. The symptoms intensified early in the treatment, and at one point I was wondering if I would be the first HT practitioner to call 911.

Within about ten minutes the severe symptoms subsided. Thirty minutes later Diane's field was totally clear, her head was clear, the breathing was normal and the headache was totally gone. The client felt normal and the lily was still sitting next to her head. At this time

I removed the lily and did a Basic Balance (Cath Webber-Martin) to stabilize the energy field. After grounding, I asked the client to stay away from lilies for two or three days to let the field adjust and stabilize. Later in the week she called to say that she went to the grocery store and spent several minutes in the flower department near the lilies with no reaction to any blooms. This was first time Diane was exposed to lily blooms in many years with no reaction. She was a happy lady.

In conclusion, it is clear that allergic reactions can be severe and even life threatening. Practitioners should be careful. In this case I knew I could remove the stimulus at any time, but that might not always be true. I feel there is a real potential for energetic intervention to heal allergic reactions.

Don Stouffer
Cincinnati, Ohio

Heart to Heart: Working with Multiple Sclerosis
I have known Randy and Helen for many years, we are good friends and we have traveled together. Helen started with multiple sclerosis in 1993 when motor and sensitivity dysfunctions started to appear. In spring, 1996 Helen became paralyzed from the mid torso to the feet. I went to see Helen in the hospital, talked about Healing Touch, and began to work with her. She has been a client since that time.

Real progress occurred with some Energetic Healing techniques later that year. I felt from the beginning that Helen's bout with the MS resulted from her son Bart (18) who committed suicide 1992. The guilt, anger and frustration were extreme, and they had a profound effect on Helen's life after 1992. The lesions on her spine are at the heart chakra. Helen's heart was broken. I could feel the pain.

I gave her several treatments and many of the physical limitations were improving. I really got to know Helen during this period, and she was now willing to work with me on the Bart suicide. The first key session started with a chakra connection to clear and balance the system. I focused energy on the lesions, lower chakras and legs since walking was better, but still not normal. I next did an Energy Field Drain and asked Helen to think of Bart and the related issues. Helen's field immediately closed. The drain was thick and gooey on the Etheric level. I could feel the pain and anger in the Astral Body, and the Ketheric template was prickly. I sensed an "energy infection" on a higher level, and I asked the Guides to take me there to drain the trauma. The energy flow was incredibly strong, and Helen said she could feel the pain leaving. The lower levels then cleared easily. The chakras were open and the aura extended several feet. The "energy infection" was gone. I next asked Helen how she would like to feel about Bart. Helen could not accept a position of love, so a feeling of "truth without guilt" was added during the replenishment phase of the treatment. The treatment ended with a full body connection and an energy blessing. Helen was now able to talk about Bart without pain and adverse emotions. She felt "peaceful and relaxed" for the first time since the trauma.

The second key treatment focused on the heart chords. During the previous treatment I observed disruption in the heart chords between Helen and Bart. All four chords were damaged and disconnected. They were all attached to Helen, but were a tangled, torn, matted knot in Helen's chest. A Heart Chakra Clearing and Balancing were used with the intention to clean and clear the heart chords. This step was done twice. After some discussion with Helen I asked Randy's spirit to be present. (He was physically at work.) His heart chakra was balanced, and his heart chords were attached to Helen and appeared very strong and healthy. The four free chords attached to Helen were attached to Bart, and melted and fused into the existing chords. I asked God and Guides to help strengthen the bond and terminated the treatment. Helen told me she is now at peace with Bart.

In the two years since these treatments Helen has been almost symptom free. She gets a few mild symptoms after periods of extreme stress, but nothing like before the treatments. She is fully functional. Her husband, Randy, does Healing Touch on her every week. I see her three or four times a year for tune-ups. Discussions of Bart do nothing to her energy field. The trauma is gone.

Don Stouffer
Cincinnati, Ohio

Healing Touch and Bipolar Disorder

Jane had a long standing history of many years of manic depression (that was not well controlled no matter what drugs or psychotherapy were used) called me about a year ago requesting HT to see if that would help her in any way with this problem. One of the difficulties was that in order to feel somewhat in balance she had to take an amount of drugs that then gave her unpleasant side effects that to her seemed as difficult to deal with as the mood swings. I saw her weekly for a few months and then we were able to transition to once a month that coincided with her monthly therapy session which was a schedule that she felt benefited her best. The primary energy treatment was chakra connection followed by mind clearing usually done in an hour time frame. Gradually over time the field would hold for longer periods of time. Initially everything was closed and the head gave off very erratic energy. She also had difficulty staying in her field and would often have it somewhere above her. Sometimes I would Unruffle her back in but often I found using the Chakra connection as the treatment where I would hold each place however long it took to feel balance rather then just a minute or two would bring her back into her field.

At this time I see her every 4-5 weeks still in conjunction with her therapy appointment and she is now off all medication. Her energy field stays in place and open from one visit to the next. She reports feeling in a balanced mood that she cannot remember ever knowing before. She has practiced some self-balancing that I taught her and recently took Level I HT because she wanted to better understand the work that has so greatly changed her life. (Note: medication weaning was done in consultation with her psychiatrist who was also following her for medical management.) At this time, because she has responded so well and her illness has been so long standing, she is comfortable with this maintenance plan. The long term goal is to see if she can eventually maintain this stability with self-balancing.

Deny Brown
Richmond, Virginia

Working with Blood Transfusion Clients

I arranged to do a healing on a friend, B. I commenced and carried out the usual treatment sequence having taken a history. I intuitively felt that she should rest for the rest of the day, and that I should see her again within days. I asked if that was possible. She said yes as she was coming into Nelson where I was going to be for the weekend. I borrowed a room in Joan Luff's house. I commenced working automatically using Energetic Healing work. I knew I was working with "something" which was coming from B which I didn't know about. It felt like mercury (quicksilver), breaking up and moving to different areas, including the floor. I couldn't contain it. After the treatment B said she felt great. I asked Joan to come into the room and together managed to clear the room and subsequently the property.

However I went out to dinner and I still had this cold feeling in my solar plexus. My host wanted me to do a healing for her and although I was not keen, I did it. The next day I was feeling quite unwell and did a lot of crying. I then discovered on the following day that my host felt the same. We met that night. I was asked to tell another HT practitioner who is a very clear channel, about this experience. The result was the following. K said the angels present wanted me to know that I could create a mesh (like gossamer web) and place this in the etheric field. I could then do the work and when I asked they (the angels) would quickly remove the web which would then contain whatever it was. They then channeled that what I had was "sorrow" which had been transfused into B at surgery many years again in England. The blood had come from two different people both who had huge levels of sorrow and had now died and realized that they needed to "reclaim" this. I asked if I could check and work with my client over the distance to ensure her clearing of this. The answer was "yes." That completed I asked if I could please clear all the people involved in this including myself and was again given an affirmative being told they would assist.

I now use this technique whenever I know a transfusion has been given, a transfusion is in progress or an organ transplant has been received. When I returned to my home some days later, I phoned B to check how she was. She said she felt "great." I explained that I had taken the liberty of doing some distance work and that she had been cleared of "sorrow which was not hers." Her immediate response was that, "I always knew it was not mine." I did NOT tell her how she had come by it as she may well need surgery again in the future and fear she does not need.

Annis Parker
Christchurch, New Zealand

Lessons and Insights:
1) An advanced practitioner frequent while they are in the middle of work will be given new techniques that are not only specific to the person being treated, but generic messages for others to benefit from.
2) If the healer is not feeling well extra precautions need to be taken to keep from passing on "garbage." This is not unlike what happens in any other situation as if we are out of sorts, or irritable we need to get clear and not pass on our unfinished business to others. It is the phenomena of a bad day at work and taking it out on the family. It is the same concept in energy work.
3) This new technique inserting a gossamer web is a concrete way to provide protection to the self and others. There are additional measures that can be taken such as bringing in a golden light, using sounding or toning, keeping the vibrations raised sufficiently to not have anything drain back into the system. The basic centering taught in HT level one is the best for beginning practitioners—going inside, asking for guidance to be clear channel for the client, connecting with the client, setting the intention and going back to the process if the energy falls.

Why I Love This Work: Hospice Care

In my first home visit to Jerry, a 52 year old recovering street person with terminal cancer of the throat, I was touched by the warmth and love that filled the small cottage overlooking Puget Sound. While his wife was at work, his sister was there as caregiver. The sister expressed concern for the wife, her exhaustion and the recently discovered breast lump. She asked if I could arrange to work on the wife at some point, too. I started to explain that hospice policy didn't permit me to treat family members unless they paid for my services, when the wife arrived home for lunch. Her need was obvious, and suddenly the rules seemed irrelevant. With an open heart, I suggested she join in the treatment by sitting in the recliner at Jerry's bedside while I worked on him, with the intent that she too, receive the healing energy. Mozart accompanied us throughout the visit—Jerry's choice.

As I began to work, I was guided to suggest that she call in any helpful spirit guides or saints to help with the healing. All I knew about the couple is that they had lived together for several years, but had only had an official marriage ceremony three weeks earlier. But the Madonna on the end table and the cross on the mantel suggested to me that someone here was Catholic, and probably open to such a concept. After the treatment, she thanked me profusely, saying she felt closer to her husband during that session than ever before. She had felt a blending of their energies in a way his illness had long prevented. Physical closeness was too painful for him. Furthermore, it turned out that she had formerly been a nun, and when she asked for spirit guides to assist, she called on the spirit of her Mother Superior, who had since died. She done her novitiate training at the same convent where our local Healing Touch practice group volunteers their services. Jerry slept soundly through the night, and then slipped into a restless unconsciousness the next day. I did another treatment a few days later, which relieved his restlessness. He died in peace before dawn the next morning.

Mary Ellis
Olympia, Washington

Working with Addictions: Women in Prison

For a little over three years now, I've been visiting the San Francisco Women's Jail. Before I began, I was told that most of the women there had been jailed for violations related to substance abuse, prostitution, and alcoholism. Now, after having visited with over two hundred women, I am inclined to say that yes they were sentenced for those offenses, but as I see it, the first cause and basic reason for their being in jail has to do with childhood trauma or wounds. One can hardly imagine the harm done to little children and babies, even before birth, by parental substance abuse and neglect, not to mention the violence of being beaten, locked in dark closets, not being fed, left alone, rejected and even raped.

One day before I became known as a "healer," I was visiting the jail and a woman asked me if I could help her. "Why, certainly, I want to be of help." I responded, "What is it?"

She explained: "Some years ago I was hacked by a big butcher knife while I lay on the floor with my small son under me to protect him. I thought we were both going to be killed. I still have nightmares about it. Every night I wake up the other women with my screaming."

I told her that I thought I could help her with a treatment called Healing Touch. I explained a little about it, that it was an ancient art, and so forth. "Next time I come to visit," I said, "I'll ask for a private room and permission to give you a treatment." Suddenly it occurred to me that she was asking for help now. Why should she have to wait? I asked if she would like to pray the Lord's Prayer with me right then, standing close to me so that I could place my hand over the center of her body. She agreed, and we prayed together. After the prayer, I assured her that I would work longer with her the next time I came, when we had a private room. She sad that she already felt better. After two treatments, she had no more nightmares, no more screaming in the middle of the night.

The other inmates notice the change right away, since they were no longer being awakened nightly, and asked her what had happened. In this way the good news of the healing spread, and soon other women came to tell me their stories and ask for a healing. They are still coming. I tell them that they are in charge of their lives, and if they really want to, they can heal. I am just the channel of God's healing light and energy. For the most part, the women I see are ready for healing. The jail has good programs for rehabilitation, like counseling, acupuncture, yoga meditation, etc., and these women take advantage of the sessions offered. Like the woman with the nightmares, they have dreadful childhood and adult experiences to deal with and heal.

One day after I became a Certified Healing Touch Practitioner and had taken advanced classes in Energetic Healing from Dr. Mary Jo Bulbrook, it occurred to me to try and heal addictions. And so I do, with apparent good results. One by one the inmates come in with "helpful talk," energy assessment, and then centering in the Divine, we begin our healing. I find that it is best to start with the healing for any physical pain using Unruffling and Pain Drain. If the person has childhood wounds, I use the Core Star Expansion. Other modalities are used as seem right, like the Hara Alignment to help the person see the reason or purpose for being on this earth. Before beginning the healing of addictions, it seems best to work on childhood wounds and subsequent traumas. In my limited experience of eleven months, using the Core Star expansion and a series of other modalities as needed does the healing of addictions most effectively. I encourage those being healed to continue their practice of what they have learned, like meditation, deep breathing, and exercise.

Treatments to the women in the jail are stepped up in time and energy. I usually visit four times a month, and generally there are six, seven, even eight women waiting for healing. The sheriff's deputies give me as much time as I need, and sometimes even go to the trouble of switching room assignments around in order to accommodate us. As I leave, I thank the deputies, who often thank me in turn for my work. Apparently they see a difference for the better in the women.

Several women I've worked with in the jail are now back in the community, pursuing various programs and living in half-way houses, so I am able to follow up on them. It is rewarding to assess their energy fields, chat with them and realize that they are on their way to recovery. From the very first sessions with each woman, I encourage follow-up treatments whenever possible to reinforce the energy field and to give moral support. This is especially important in cases of addition. For where there is no follow-up at times there is relapse.

I am pleased to report that one woman, my first addiction client, was placed in a halfway house in my parish eleven months ago. While living there she received training to become a medical assistant, and she now has a job. She is a lector at church each Sunday. She has also taken Healing Touch on a partial scholarship and is practicing it in her halfway house.

Two more Healing Touch students are applying to be volunteers at the jail adding to the foundation that I put in place. My prayer is that healing may be available to the most vulnerable and then spread outward to you world. It has been an honor to be of help in healing addictions of women in prison!

Sister Barbara Cavanaugh, RSM
San Francisco, California

Easing His Pain: Loving Him to Death

Intake: Henry is a 69 year old widower with end stage head cancer with the left side of his head very affected. The cancer has broken through the skin and is slowly progressing downward and outward to the left eye area. The tissue is very necrotic, odorous, and hideous. Henry had been living alone for six years. He and his wife had been separated a few years before she died. Henry was a very private, independent man, stubborn in his ways. He had two grown married nieces who were his lifeline.

Henry developed a head sore over a year ago and paid little attention to it until it became infected. He refused to see a doctor, wanting to care for it himself. He lived in great poverty with little running water only in the kitchen. His sore grew larger and Henry would try to bandage it as best he could. He didn't want anyone "messing with him." Eventually it became unmanageable and his nieces brought him to the doctor. He was diagnosed with cancer and ended up in hospice care. After time, the dire poverty of his living conditions and no running water created a situation where our home staff could not give optimal care. Neither Henry nor his two nieces were able to care for the wound. Due to its severity, the cancer became unmanageable. Working with the social worker, his two nieces, and the doctor, Henry was offered a room at our "Hospice Home" of Burlington, NC. It is a six-bed free standing, non-profit home for the terminally ill supported by an all-volunteer hospice league.

It took great pains and coaxing for Henry to leave the security of his home, saying he would only give it a try. Silently, we all thanked God, knowing this was the place for him and we knew we would be "loving him to death". We understood how difficult and scared he was to be uprooted. He came to us on a Monday morning, the first week of June, 1998. As a Certified Nursing Assistant, I was briefed along with the other staff and a care plan was implemented for Henry. The first few days were challenging, ordering supplies. The odor was permeating the house, which embarrassed Henry and kept him in his room. The wound site was hideous to see and clean. Somewhere, we were told, were maggots inside. The dressings had to be changed twice daily. I worked second shift 3:30 p.m.-12:00 a.m. The Licensed Practical Nurse working with me, Ann, had personally been healed of a hand injury with Healing Touch when I first began my studies. She knows I use it much on our shift and is supportive.

The first night Ann and I did Henry's dressing, he watched our every reaction. We worked very gently through pleasant conversation and assured him of our love and support. He was so grateful. We said our good nights, left the room sick at heart and to our stomachs at the sight and the smell. Though we see much cancer, it is never easy to overcome our emotions at the hideousness of it. I went home and prayed all night for Henry, for guidance to help this man and the next morning work up with a Healing Touch plan to explain to Ann. We asked Henry if he would be open to it. We could all learn from the Divine to help Henry and us to manage this head wound. I gave Henry a brief explanation of Healing Touch, explaining it very simply through a Christ picture Henry loved in his room. He brought it from home and had it a long time. The white light surrounding the Christ scenes in his picture was an area that surrounds all our bodies, we just can't see it yet. Some call it God force, some call it life force. I have been taught to ask for guidance and to place my hands inside at different levels and in different places to help people with pain. Would he like me to help him in this way? Henry became very thoughtful and agreed.

The Healing Touch plan was directed to: a) minimize pain during and after debriding, b) stop bleeders (very common) during debriding, c) eliminate odor, and d) enhance quality of life. I held the light to create a sacred space to work. The rotting flesh was cleared, irrigated, and covered with a clean dressing. Bleeders were quickly stopped with Ultrasound. The 45 minute procedure was done night after night in an effort to ease his pain. Henry said he never felt hurt. By August he was a changed man, free of odor, and able to get about and spend quality time with family.

I stayed at his side as much as possible, helping him journey into the light. On November 25, one month before Christmas, Henry died with great ease, peace, and surrounded by love. Ann and I were at his side and at his last breath, he opened his good eye, looked out, smiled, and left.

Thank you Henry, Healing Touch, and the Divine. All gifts to me.

Joan Lallier
Burlington, North Carolina

Instructor's Note: When Joan presented this case study at her HT Level IIIB, the completion of her practitioner's training in HT, there wasn't a dry eye in the room. The love and caring was truly the presence of the Divine operating through her as an instrument of love. I told Joan it was clear to me that when I die I want to have her care for me as it would be the highest one could ask for. This experience exemplifies what the work is all about. Joan and her teammate were angels sent by God to ease his pain. It reinforces to me the importance of their role. CNA and LPN titles don't do justice to what I witnessed. I hereby bestow on them (if I really could I would) a new title, AWH—Angels Working Here. (Mary Jo Bulbrook)

An Unexpected Turn

Over the years I have facilitated many healing treatments and have never ceased to be amazed at some of the remarkable things, which have happened. One that stands out for me, was the story of Mandy Lewis. Mandy, a 28 year old single woman, came to me on the recommendation of a Tarot reader who felt she was in need of some healing work. Mandy was suffering from a potentially life threatening condition called Lupus (a chronic, usually lifelong, potentially fatal auto-immune disease involving joints, skin and organs of the body) and was in considerable pain. Due to the debilitating effects of this condition her emotional state was very fragile and she was quite depressed. Mandy felt traditional medicine wasn't helping her and decided to try energy based healing to see if it could assist her. This was the first time she had ever experienced anything outside of the traditional mainstream medical treatment and didn't really believe in "this sort of thing" as she put it. However, she had reached the point of desperation.

From the first treatment her improvement was immediate. There was instant relief from the pain, her emotional state began to improve and she started to feel this condition was at last going to be manageable. Mandy herself experienced the most remarkable thing. She saw colors during the healing process! This amazed her and led to the realization of another dimension she had not seriously considered before.

We began a healing program which was to span several months interspersed with bouts of ill health as the Lupus continued to debilitate the physical body. She came to realize that even though she had this condition, there was a way of controlling her emotional and mental well-being. Energy based healing was proving to be very effective in controlling pain as well as helping emotion and mental well-being. I worked under guidance using a combination of Healing Touch, Esoteric Healing, and Intuitive Healing. I myself saw many different images and light of differing colors being placed throughout the body and organs as the treatments progressed. Mandy always received relief from her pain after each of these treatments.

During one of the treatments I was told, "The source of the problem was in the brain—something was misfiring." I didn't understand this at the time but noted it and continued on with the treatments.

The last time I worked with Mandy was after she had been in hospital and had surgery after a very severe flare up of the Lupus. The surgery had proved to be a complete failure and left her with more problems than she had before. Her pain had also become unbearable, but she came to me for a treatment, as she felt sure it would give her relief. I was to experience a very different treatment this time myself. The energy felt totally different to me. The energy at the base chakra was almost nonexistent and had what I described as, "an almost ethereal quality" to it. While holding this centre, I saw what looked like a snake, it was spiraling up the centre of her body. I was told, "Ida was missing. The Kundalini had been raised artificially in a past life and was damaged through wrong practices. The soul was seeking expression and this vital piece was missing."

The work done during this healing was to aid in the repair and reconnection of the Kundalini on the soul level. I had a sense of something very important happening but was simply unable to comprehend much of the work being done during this healing. While I was holding the ajna (brow) centre, I was told, "This healing work is the greatest service we can do for a fellow soul."

This treatment was so different from all others I had facilitated before, not only on this client, but on the many which I have performed over the years. In hindsight I was to understand why through the unexpected turn that took place.

We made an appointment for the following week but a few days later Mandy's mother was to ring and tell me Mandy had died suddenly from an aneurysm in the brain (an aneurysm is a dilatation and weakening of a blood vessel that often goes undetected until a major problem occurs such as a stroke or rupture often leading to death) that had gone undetected by the medical profession. Now I understand the meaning of the message, "the source of the problem was in the brain."

The doctor told Mandy's mother, the aneurysm had nothing to do with the Lupus and was most unexpected. It did however answer some of those questions for me about why the last treatment I did was so different. In hindsight, I believe what I was experiencing during these treatments, were energetic interventions, which assisted in the repair of the damaged Kundalini. This would allow the Soul to express itself free of this impediment in future incarnations. Finally I gained an understanding of some of those things which had baffled me during the healing treatments. This was both a privilege and honor to be allowed to participate in this sacred part of a person's life.

Janeece Kelsall
Geelong, Victoria, Australia

Healing the Present, Releasing the Past

As a practitioner of Healing Touch, Spiritual Healing, and Esoteric Healing with more years than I intend to divulge spent with this challenging, and exciting work, I can attest to the constant learning curve and eye-popping, roller-coaster ride of experiences involved. There are a host of stories waiting to be told, here is but one.

Several years ago, while part of a complementary therapy centre, it was my pleasure to meet Josephine. Entering my office somewhat shyly and nervously, I was immediately struck by her acute pallor and gaunt, thin figure; her pretty face masked by sadness, dark rings round her eyes. She sat down seeming uneasy to be in what must have felt like unfamiliar territory. We chatted slowly about this and that and on inquiring how she had came to seek the form of health care, she replied, "Mum said I had to." I then realized by some further remarks, that I knew Jo's mum, a fellow health care worker in a large hospital nearby, giving us some common ground upon which we could build. Once this was established Jo began to relax.

I proceeded to explain how I worked using Healing Touch entwined with Spiritual Healing. She said she felt quite comfortable with this. Jo explained she has been diagnosed as having an "eating disorder" which had bothered her for all of her young life of 24 years. All diagnostic efforts had failed to find any cause for her problems, which was basically, that she was unable to swallow solids. Jo existed on fluids and was even having difficulty with them now. The whole situation had become impossible and she was in constant fear of choking. To make matters worse, she had a small child and was becoming paranoid (her description) about her child doing the same thing (i.e. choking on food) and of a sense of being powerless to help.

I asked if she was able to pinpoint something that had happened and might be related to her condition. She related briefly about attending a "Spiritual Church." In hindsight something within her energy system must have been triggered at that visit.

As we talked, it became more obvious not only was Jo racked by fears of all kinds including the fear of making mistakes. She openly stated that she greatly resented the responsibility of raising a child as a single parent. She was paralyzed by concern about what others thought. In her words, she said, "I have lost my old fun loving self. Life is no longer fun nor is it a pleasure. I feel like curling up and dying."

It seemed time to begin to restructure and repair whatever the need was in her energy system. The first treatment consisted of a general energy body (auric) balance. Additional attention was given to an area, proven in practice to release fears, increase vitality with particular attention being paid to the throat area (the area of greatest immediate distress), where much clearing and balancing was done, a simple and straightforward treatment.

A week later, Jo returned for a second treatment. She strode into the room with a beaming smile, brighter, animated and much more self assured. She related how she felt more positive, was eating better and even socializing again! This was a very pleasing development.

Without further conversation, we proceeded with the second treatment. This time Healing Touch was woven with Spiritual Healing or guided work. Much clearing of the field was achieved using specific Healing Touch techniques which facilitated healing on a deep level. I was directed to implement a powerful energy circuit for releasing past life trauma. Much guided assistance was the "order of the day." I was "shown" a past life trauma which lay at the foot of this young lady's difficulties today. I was also advised to inform her of them and of what had transpired, at the end of the session.

During this treatment Jo relaxed deeply. I waited for her to come back to full awareness before disturbing her. Over a cup of coffee, we discussed our shared experiences (Jo said she saw certain inexplicable scenes). When the conversation presented the appropriate opportunity, I related to her the following information that came to me to see if it had any relevance to her: "As a young man of 24, a Lancer in the Light Horse fighting in the Boar War, riding full pelt during a charge, you were accidentally struck across the throat with a gun barrel by a comrade in arms, breaking the windpipe and stopping all ability to continue."

Jo looked at me, went a little pale and said, "Yes, it's OK, it makes sense." Then she said, "I saw some of that, that's what I was seeing!" Then she asked, "What country had the Boar War been fought?" I said, "It was in Africa." "Yes," said Jo, "that does make sense. Guess what? My whole throat problem became intolerable after reading the book *The Power of One* (set in Africa) and another book on Africa!" Needless to say we were both rather quiet for a while.

Upon arrival the following week, a "new woman" greeted me. She was glowing and happily spoke about how good life was again! She now had a job at long last in great surroundings, was able to eat and drink almost anything and generally coping with life and her young child in a normal and relaxed manner. Her final treatment was one to consolidate and balance her renewed vigor.

Now several years later Jo has not looked back and leads a full life, with good health and an advancing career. This is a dramatic case illustrates one of the most common causes of often unsuspected and unrecognized baffling health problems which are resistant to treatment. It is an essential area of clearing which will feature more and more in the future. Not in all similar cases is it necessary nor advisable to inform the person of the past life trauma apprehended. It is sufficient to clear it, enabling them to get on with this life without further incapacitating restrictions.

Footnote: the acute choking problem became exacerbated at the exact age in which the past life throat injury was sustained. This same correlation of onset of specific symptoms or aggravation of a problem has been found in numerous such cases encountered.

Cath Webber-Martin
Queenscliff, Victoria, Australia

Panic Attacks and Anorexia

Judy was a very thin, listless female in her twenties when she came to the center to see me. She described a fairly recent history of panic attacks in which her heart pounded, she felt the need to get out of whatever situation she was in, and just couldn't handle it any more. She had heard of my work and was willing to try whatever I had to offer.

I am a registered nurse, formerly an intensive care nurse, a certified holistic nurse, and have had a private practice and Holistic Health Center since my certification in HT in 1993. For more than ten years I have been doing something called Spirit Release in which we help trapped souls who may be in the clients body or aura return to the Light. It is not unlike a very gentle exorcism. In the past, it is not something I talked about a lot. I mention my background because I attempt to maintain a very professional orientation to the general public so they will feel safe in coming for holistic treatment. I can hardly say, "For the past few years I've found it really helps to do an exorcism for those symptoms as part of your Healing Touch session." So, I gently integrate the spirit release into the session. The patient is seldom aware of anything different.

It was this that I did for Judy. I had her take off her shoes and lay on the massage table. I covered with a light cotton blanket, centered myself, and asked for the presence, guidance and assistance of the God and her guides. I asked, in my mind, for St. Michael the Archangel to come with his golden net, the whales, dolphins and fishes and take to the Light anything that is not for the highest and best good of this client. (St. Michael uses a giant golden net along with the whales, dolphins and fishes to gently pull the net from beneath the client's feet all the way through their body, up and out the crown. Anything that he has picked up is securely encapsulated and taken to the Light.) Physically, I feel for this net with my hand, asking to feel where the congestion of any trapped souls might be. It usually goes pretty slowly. If the net seems to be stuck, I send more energy to that spot, and ask for Gods help to release this trapped energy.

When I got to Judy's abdomen, the net would not move. I said, "Judy, do you know how you are always picking stuff up from people?" She nodded. "Well, why don't you just release it all now. Just release and let go so you no longer have to carry their burdens. That's good. Just release." Soon, the net was moving freely and traveled on up through her body and out her crown. I asked St. Michael to come again this time with a smaller gauge net. He did. I followed it gently through without any major stops. I then did a normal, simple HT treatment to balance and clear any remaining "normal" congestion. After the treatment Judy said she felt fine, although a little empty inside. I advised her to keep herself full of light. I suggested that she just touch her naval and imagine it was turning a halogen light on inside. (She really had no language or experience with energy work and didn't know how to fill herself with light.)

The following week Judy returned for her follow up visit. She was animated as she settled down in the chair for our intake. Not only had she not had any more panic attacks, but also *she was no longer anorexic*! This was profound for her and for me, as she had not shared that she was suffering with anorexia. Sometimes, when people die, they don't find their way to the light and take up residence in and around someone who is a friendly receiver, or has some of those same tendencies. These lost souls then can influence the "hosts'" physical and emotional/mental life. Evidently while doing the Golden Net, St. Michael had removed and taken to the light not only the energies that were causing her to have panic attacks, but also the one who had died of anorexia. I referred her for counseling for the residual habits and underlying feelings that may have initiated the attraction of these particular energies in the first place. I did not see her again.

Kathy Sinnett
Detroit, Michigan

The Importance of History in Healing

As a Certified Holistic Nurse and a massage therapist practicing Healing Touch, I see a variety of clients in my private practice. Many are referred by physicians. Mrs. M was referred to me by a Board Certified Internist for Healing Touch and massage to release stress due to a "broken heart" from a death.

When Mrs. M arrived she was with her husband, a vigorous 79 year old man, who was a strong advocate of complementary medicine. He expressed much anger and hostility toward the medical profession calling them "greedy." He further stated he was a strong advocate of alternative medicine and began to relate very informed information. "This is a switch I though smugly For once, an enlightened person who understands complementary therapies."

Mrs. M was an attractive, graying, well preserved woman about a decade younger than her husband. She sat subdued in the waiting room chair not able to get in a word. She continuously nodded her head in agreement as her husband continued to expound. "We are both professional, accomplished, wealthy and intelligent," he said loudly in an intimidating voice. "We both know a lot about alternative medicine from reading and the Internet."

I was not intimidated. My only problem was to get Mr. M to stop talking and get Mrs. M alone. For her husband said that he wanted to come in and watch what I did. I thought it possible that Mr. M was reacting out of fear and I took a risk. I insisted that I see his wife alone or I would not see her at all. He was shocked. And I quickly asked Mrs. M to follow me back to my private office which she did.

History showed Mrs. M to be an active, physically fit woman. She tearfully related the story of her 37 year old son's illness and death six months ago following a rapid, fulminating cancer. She said, "Her heart was aching since that time." Further history elicited the onset of severe chest pain upon sweeping the lanai following cooking dinner for 60 guests the previous day! "That is enough to make anyone have chest pain," I thought to myself.

Mrs. M's breathing was within normal limits, her skin was dry, her nail beds were pale, her pulse was rapid and thready, her color very tan. Her Blood Pressure was slightly elevated. She had no pain at this time. An energy assessment elicited a severe denseness over the heart area. It felt like concrete. A sensation of little sparks bounced off my palms. As I passed over the heart area again to clear it, Mrs. M began to cry and process her son's death. Holding her hand and listening I began to stroke her arm lightly. I listened with compassion and sent a lovely pink color to her heart

After she finished her story she seemed to be less afraid and I continued with my history taking. Where was the pain? What did it feel like? How long did it last? When did the pain occur? All the questions that I could think of, for I was intuiting that the "concrete" and "sparks" were something more than grief.

Her answers were not significant. "Have you ever had an EKG?" I asked still probing. "Yes," she said. "When and what did it show?" I continued. "Well, they said I needed a stress test, but my husband won't let me get one as he said that the doctors are after our money. He said everyone knows that my heart pain is from the loss of Brian, our son and I need to see a holistic person."

"Yes, that may be true," I said gently, "but before I will see you again you need to see a cardiologist." Mrs. M began to sob, then said, "At last! Someone who believes me, believes that my pains are real. Now you have to convince my husband."

"Oh, boy! This is my lucky day," I thought. "Now I have to argue against complementary therapies." Donning my white jacket for professional support and slinging my stethoscope around my neck, I left the room immediately. I informed Mr. M that his wife needed to see a cardiologist at once! He was shocked and said, "But I thought you were one of those other kind of nurses."

"I am. I am a Certified Holistic Nurse," I replied, "but you cannot throw the baby out with the bath water." I then explained that I thought his wife was having more than heart pains from grief and that I would hold him responsible if anything happened to her if he did not consult a cardiologist. Tough words for a tough man!

"Okay," he said in a confrontational manner. "I am going to do what you said but we are not coming back here, that is for sure. The doctor said you would do a Healing Touch and a massage." When Mrs. M came out we briefly discussed my findings. "Come on, let's go," he said gruffly. "I'm going to take you to a heart doctor and then find you a good massage therapist." They left the office quickly and I documented the visit and faxed it to the Internist's office. I didn't hear anything for over two weeks. As is my custom, I called Mrs. M for a follow-up. She answered the phone.

"How are you?" I asked sincerely. "Oh, I'm fine. I had heart surgery two days after I saw you. I had four blocked arteries to my heart. Two were completely blocked." I was delighted with the news and said a quick prayer of thanks that I followed my nursing assessment skills. I told her how happy I was that she went to see the cardiologist. We said our good-byes when she added. "Oh, Barbara, thank you so much. I won't see you again. My husband won't let me. He wants me to see a real alternative therapist."

Barbara Harris
Osprey, Florida

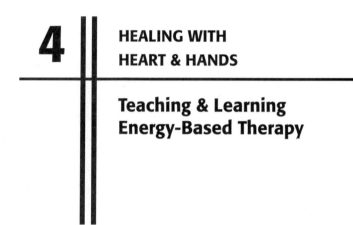

4 HEALING WITH HEART & HANDS

Teaching & Learning Energy-Based Therapy

Energetic Healing Salutation
Dredging the depths of my small self,
Wounded fragments found there, then
Surfaced in dedicated intention,
Becomes, in each encounter
A mighty energetic relinquishment
To the clearing of my united
Self-with-self
That brings clarity
To my life
And true life's purpose.

Energetic Healing from the Heart.
Given, and received.

Anne Boyd
Augusta, Georgia

Teaching Persons with Special Needs

In South Africa in 1996 I taught my first blind student in a class of six people. It was the first Healing Touch class in South Africa. I knew that it would be challenging for me, but I wanted to measure up to the call.

I became so aware of the things seeing-eye people take for granted. As I held my hands out and said "do this" or "hold your hands this way," I realized Brian could not know what to do. Everything I did had to be evaluated as to if it was understandable to someone who could not see. Believe me, it was a challenge, especially since no one else knew anything about HT and therefore couldn't assist me with classroom dynamics. So there I was, doing a juggling act totally stressed as to the importance of being understood by others. Not unlike the young man I was serving experiences most of the time!

I was so pleased with my efforts because once I let go I took it on as a challenge to be clear and helpful. I learned some new ways to present material through the sense of tactile expression. I learned how to teach honoring all clients and sharing with them through conquering their disability.

I also learned patience and tolerance of those who are different. My reward was when Brian came back after the first day and reported he had treated both his grandmother and grandfather who paid for him to come to class! I realized then, that this young man would make it work for him. I was proud to be part of his teaching and proud of myself for overcoming my prejudices of questioning the need to limit healing.

Another experience I wish to report actually happened to Donna Duff. One of her students had a partial arm and hand on one side. When asked if she could participate, Donna said of course. During the exchanges Donna watched with pride that the woman was totally engrossed in the healing and the recipient reported "feeling" two hands on her!

The last example I want to report is about a beautiful woman who had been paralyzed by a car accident and was in a wheel chair. I was teaching a HT Level IIB in Virginia when she was a student in the classroom. Her needs presented different challenges for the teacher. I also watched in amazement as all of the techniques were done with her hands held towards the client as she could not reach the positions.

The clients reported very profound experiences—no different than any others!

I learned the importance of making healing available to all people if it is their choice to follow this path.

Mary Jo Bulbrook
Carrboro, North Carolina

Lessons and Insights:
1) Those with special needs present challenges both in the class-room and outside as they move to practice what they have learned. Helping them through these difficulties brings rewards not only to the special needs student but also to those who are served by them as well as the teacher!
2) The giving of care by special needs students' produces results similar to any other student.
3) We have an obligation as teachers to open our knowledge to those who have challenges in learning.
4) The boost in the special needs person's self-esteem as they learn new things and overcome hurdles is rich beyond measure.
5) Accept special needs students as the gift from God that they are, as they have much to teach each of us!

Blue Bubbles of Healing

At a recent Healing Touch Workshop, Bonnie, one of the partici-pants shared this story with the group after Pain Drain had been demonstrated. She had learned the technique from a friend and decided to use it during a Reiki treatment with a man who had an old painful shoulder injury. During her treatment she encouraged him to be open to receive. As he relaxed and closed his eyes, he began picturing himself sucking energy through a straw as he experienced the heat of her hands. When she placed her left hand on his shoulder he visualized the pain leaving the area.

After the treatment he shared that during the treatment he began to visualized blue bubbles cascading down into her body with one going into her heart and the next going into his injury. The sensation was one of healing and connectedness. They both realized that the blue bubble vision probably occurred when she moved her left hand from the wound to a position above to receive light healing energy from the universe and placed her right hand on the injury. No wonder she decided to take Healing Touch and use this for friends. She had a wonderful experience of healing from the heart and he was relieved of his pain!

Bernie Clarke
Olympia, WA

Lessons and Insights:
1) Doing the work is what is needed rather than talking about it for energy based healing sells itself.
2) Pain Drain is very effective in relieving pain of all kinds. Those who take the time to "experience" the treatment will often have extra sensory awareness.
3) Even when as a healer you are not totally aware of what is happening, the client can describe extraordinary occurrences. Being open to this dimension can be yield exciting new levels of awareness.
4) Healer and client are in a mutual co-creation of realty. They are intimately connected that transcends traditional descriptions of client/healer relationships.

Opening My Mind to Healing Touch

When I first heard of Healing Touch I had no idea what to expect. I was very interested in finding out how it worked, but I was also very skeptical. I decided to take the Healing Touch Level I class to learn more about it. I knew I needed to have an open mind to truly get anything from the class, but I still had my reservations going into it.

When the class started, everyone was feeling or seeing things that I wasn't. I was having a hard time believing in it, so my mind was not letting me experience it. However, that all changed when we started working with the chakras. I could not believe that we had seven different energy sources in our bodies that could move a pendulum clockwise. I was positive that my instructor was moving it with her hand. However, in the class you experience everything hands-on. Therefore, when it was my turn to test the chakras, I refused to move my hand in any way. I was determined to prove to myself that it was not real. But then something amazing happened, it moved. My pendulum started rotating and the circle became bigger and bigger as

I held it over the chakra. I was astonished!

That became the turning point for me. From then on, I looked at the teachings in the class with an open mind. I started experiencing things that I had never felt before. I shared many new experiences with the people in my class and left with a new feeling of belief and strength. That class not only taught me the techniques of Healing Touch, but also helped open my mind.

Mandy Chvala
Midlothian, Virginia

Seeing Things from a Different Point of View

Before I share my story with you, I think I need to give a little background is in order. I think that understanding who I am, and where I came from, will help some of the disbeliever's out there. My name is Bill, and I am one of Mary Jo's sons. I have grown up having Energetic Healing and Healing Touch as a part of my life. Different techniques have been used on my brothers and I our whole lives, and only recently have I learned what has been going on all this time.

I don't think I ever really truly believed in what my mother was doing. She even did healings on me. I had personally witnessed some unbelievable healing events take place when I was younger. Still, I did not give energy work a chance. I had never tried to understand what she was doing, and what was happening when she did it. I felt better after every session, but never had the foresight to understand why. It really is not a very hard concept to grasp, once you have it explained. All you have to do is put down your guard and listen. I think my reservations stem from society, and the pressure put on us to only deal with traditional medicine. This type of work was seen as quackery in its early stages, like when I was growing up, because it was just being reinvented. No one had ever seen it before. The truth is, before modern medicine, this was the only type of healing there was. People were very against any type of new medical technique at first too, but as they saw the evidence, and experienced it working for themselves, it became mainstream. The problem was that in the process of discovering medicine, energy work and other types of healing were forgotten. Today, energy work is being more and more accepted as people see the results. Society is finally putting down its guard and learning the true power of this work.

I originally took this class as a way to better answer questions about Healing Touch since I am the business manager of my mothers company, Healing Touch Partnerships. Here I am, working around this energy concept every day and blindly strutting along like it is simply an ordinary job. What I didn't know was that taking this class would change my whole outlook on things, although I think mom had this in mind the whole time. Mothers are funny like that. They can make you do something that you don't really want to do, knowing that afterwards you really wanted to do it, and just didn't know it yet. I had been accepting the work more and more as I was submersed in the business full time, but still never believed. I knew that there had to be something to it, though, and I convinced my girlfriend and one of my best friends to take the class with me. I thought that in case the class was really boring, at least I would have someone I knew to share in my misery with me. I did have an open mind though, I think it is important to keep an open mind about everything, and I made it clear to my friends that they should too. I knew that at least having an open mind would let me understand why this affects others so powerfully. So here I am, the son of one of the pioneers in energy work, having previously witnessed its potential, even having it effectively performed on me, and I still went into the class with reservations. All your reservations disappear with your first discovery, the first time you physically feel energy.

The class begins with some background, of course, but you jump in, right away, and experience energy for yourself. You learn what an aura feels like. You also learn right off that everyone's aura feels different even though there are many similar qualities. I felt the energy right away, possibly because I had grown up with it. But after that first experience, the class was awesome. You learn of many different techniques, but the story I want to share with you stems from the later part of the class when doing the Chakra Connection, and especially the Chakra Spread.

I had the good fortune of taking this class with my girlfriend, and unknowingly at the time, this enhanced the experience even more. The Chakra Connection is two people sharing themselves in a way that you have not shared yourself before. You blend energetically, and it is one of the most peaceful, loving feelings I have ever encountered. You feel like you are the only two people on earth. The hard part to explain is that at the same time, you sense the other pairs in the room who are doing the same thing, and feel connected to them as well. Throughout this whole experience, you couldn't care less about your big test last week, the huge project you have due at work tomorrow, the fact that you have been sick all-month, none of this matters. You are submersed in the moment. You feel more alive then you have ever felt, and you are sharing it with others who love it just as much. People always say that you are most alive when closest to death. That is the reason why we skydive, go white-water rafting, play sports, get in front of a crowd. When doing these things we are living in the present. It is the only time we are not thinking about the future or the past. The fact that we are living for that exact moment is what makes these experiences so great. This same reason is why the connection is such a powerful experience. You feel more alive then you have ever felt.

Immediately after this revelation that you and all the others in the class had, you talk about your personal experiences with one another. The best part of the class was sharing what each person was feeling, and learning that they were all seeing similar things too. You share how great the Chakra Connection was and you are already mesmerized. You now learn one of the sacred techniques, the Chakra Spread, and learn that you have only sipped from the healing cup. Everyone is in this state of bliss, and now you and the same partner really open up to one another, all without having spoken a single word. There is no talking, only some background music. I personally am a music lover, so having a tune to help you get lost in yourself is wonderful. I say get lost in yourself because that is the best way I can describe what happens.

This is a technique that completely opens up your energy field. It is a sacred technique used commonly for people going through a major change in their life and for those who are about to die. It is sacred because it is too powerful to use on people who are not comfortable enough around one another. I was on the receiving end first. I was lying on my back on a table, feeling very relaxed and peaceful with some nice music playing, and the technique began. There is no talking and the giver needs to be careful not to disturb the receiver. Your whole energy field is slowly, methodically opened up. My experience was that I felt my body do some really strange things. I was almost scared because I have never felt anything remotely like this before. All of my limbs went a little numb, but it was more like I was half floating. My chest stayed on the table, but the rest of me was three feet above the table. The giver stretches your energy out and I felt myself becoming three feet taller, and on the next pass ten feet taller. I saw darkness all around at this point and this was perhaps what was a little bit scary for me. Then out of nowhere, my limbs that were floating now felt pressed against the table, and my chest was thrown up almost in a jerk. There was a massive flow of white light darting out of it in the process. I could not believe what was happening to me. It was the greatest sense of relief, yet I don't know what I was being relieved from. I guess everything that has built up inside me over the years, but I was damn happy to be relieved of it. There was all of this white light flowing out of my chest, my body was thrown back and forward at the same time, and I felt very content. The flow stopped and I was in awe. Then it happened again, and also a third time. I was just thinking, wow! This experience is hard to put into words. It is like trying to describe to someone what it feels like to be in love. It is something to experience for one's self. I opened up my eyes and looked over at my girlfriend and asked, "So was I floating six feet above the table or what?" She said that I never moved a muscle.

Now it was my turn to be the giver. I performed the technique, hoping that Mandy would have as powerful of an experience as I did. I felt myself opening and stretching her energy as I went through the whole process. I finished and still was careful not to disturb her as I stepped back and just watched. I cannot believe what I saw. First, a small beam of white light came out of her cheek. This beam of light moved up to her left eye and sat there for a second and then I saw something that I really can't believe. It was like my eyes were playing tricks on me. She was perfectly still, but the image of her started moving around in kind of a figure eight pattern, then it was not really moving in any kind of pattern, just moving around at will, never getting more than three inches away from her body. I looked out into the hall at my instructor with my jaw dropped, and she only smiled. I looked back and the image was still moving around. It slowly stabilized back on her body, and the beam of light dissipated. She opened up her eyes and asked, "Where did I go?" I told her that she didn't go anywhere, and that she hardly moved. She said, "Well then, what happened?" I said, "You tell me, I'm not even going to tell you what I saw yet!"

When everybody finished, the class gathered to again share experiences with one another. I was on cloud nine. I felt great walking out of that room. My other friend was amazed at the look on my face and could not wait to hear my story. I shared my story first. Then, as I looked around the room at everybody and listened to them share their stories, I noticed something else that's difficult to put into words. Everyone was more "there" than the rest of the things in the room. Everyone had a glow around them, but it was more than that. It was like everything else was out of focus, although it was perfectly in focus, and the people just seemed to be more *there*. I felt like a child looking around at everything for the very first time. When everyone was done sharing their stories, I just had to tell the class that everyone was glowing. They all seemed to know exactly what I was talking about.

We were asked not to discuss what may happen with this technique, since the experience is different for everyone and may not happen in a profound way for some. I had to tell my story though, because I want everyone I know to be able to experience something like this. I am currently organizing a class for my friends and family. I hope that with our prior knowledge of one another, the new class will be even more powerful than my first Level I class. Whatever you get out of this story and the others in this book, remember that it is most important to look at life with an open mind. Even if this is not the answer to your life, it will greatly help in your quest.

Bill Bulbrook
Carrboro, North Carolina

Physical Pain Transference

During an Energetic Healing class (Clearing the Internal Self), while Helen was doing Energy Field Drain and Replenishment, she experienced intense discomfort and pain in the back around the kidney area that lasted throughout the healing session. At the end of the session Helen asked me, "Is this normal?" I answered, "No," and began to ask questions about what happened to her. I asked the client if she was working on releasing fear. The client said that she was. I then asked Helen, the healer, if she also had issues around fear. She quickly said, "Yes." I told her this issue is why she couldn't process or fully clear what happened to her. It is as if the client's energy became blocked within Helen, the healer, and she became blocked within the self. I have found from experience that pain in the kidneys is related to the emotion of fear.

Mary Jo Bulbrook
Carrboro, North Carolina

Lessons and Insights:
1) If you experience discomfort while healing, it is important to identify if you have taken on the blocked energy from the client. This can only happen if it could be related to your unfinished business and you do not center and ground properly.
2) The energy clears quickly for the healer as the intervention is applied because the healer is "in relationship" with the client and is a channel for both to heal.
3) To identify if the energy is just "passing through" as you clear the client, ask inside the self the following statement, "If this is not part of my issue, please let the energy pass through."
4) It is a gift of co-creation with clients that we can be cleared of our issues while working on others. If you have problems identifying what was done, it is expected that the healer go to a mentor for help in identifying what was going on and how to work through things.
5) Energy work is very powerful and offers rich opportunities for learning as we go along. As we give, we receive. As we receive, we give. Creating the reciprocal process is very healing and prevents healer burnout.

Triggering Residual Pain from Physical Injury
During the teaching of Energy Field Drain and Replenishment, which is a technique in Energetic Healing Program, Part I (Clearing the Internal Self), the following experience occurred.

Jane was giving care to Cathy during class. As I observe Jane's technique, it looked to me that her hand was not in the right position. It was as if she was riding on top of the energy. I moved over to her and gently reposition her hand into the correct place. Immediately Jane experienced pain up her arm and the client experienced shooting intense pain out the left leg.

I stayed and coached Jane through this, as it was an "unusual occurrence." I instructed her to slow down the movement of pulling energy from the bottom of the foot chakra. As she did this, the client reported that the throbbing pain stopped. I was guided to assist with the healing and placed my hand on the back of the spine. As I did this, the client stated she had a fall three months ago and damaged her coccyx. Although it did not hurt anymore until now, the pain was excruciating, as if she had just fallen.

I asked if the problem she had worked on healing in the earlier part of the class had at its root, issues with emotions. She said, "Yes." I also asked the healer (Jane) if she also had problems with emotions, and said yes as well. What had transpired is that the healer perceived at some level the pain and was unable to access it because it mimicked her own unresolved emotional issues.

Lessons and Insights:
1) Physical pain can have a residual energy pain response that mimics the original pain. Once triggered it may behave as the original physical pain.
2) Healers with the same or similar unresolved issues as the client may not be able to access the deeper problem and/or help with the healing of the problem.
3) It is as if the physical pain was triggered through transference and felt in the hands of the healer.
4) People are guided to work together to help each other work out their issues.

Mary Jo Bulbrook
Carrboro, North Carolina

Changing the Course of Gerry's Life

While teaching a HT Level IIIA in Durham, NC in August 1993 one of the participants introduced themselves as HIV positive. This was the first time I had someone in one of my classes struggling with HIV. I watched to see how the class and I were to deal with being confronted with our issues/processes in working with HIV. The student was Gerry Mitchell. As I looked at his energy I found a very handsome man that was very powerful yet I could tell his light was dim compared to what it could be and probably had been. I also suspected that he had more of a story to tell than he was telling. The class accepted Gerry and all things went smoothly.

While I was sharing one of the many stories I often talk about in classes from my experiences of taking Healing Touch worldwide, I told that class I was planning to take a group of people to Australia and New Zealand the next year in October/November 1994. Gerry came up to me and said his angels said that he needs to go with me. I smiled and said that I would love to have him accompany me and would keep him posted of the plans. It is now a year later and again in August at the same site and I am now teaching HT Level IIIB. Gerry is there again and much stronger in energy than the year before. His eyes sparkled and he was full of experiences to share and excitement over what had been happening to him.

As I again talked about the group going to Australia and New Zealand, he came up to me and said with conviction, "I do need to go on the tour to Australia and New Zealand." I said, "Sure." While deep in my heart, I wondered how I would cope having this additional stress. Having someone with compromised health keeping up with the demanding pace we were going to have, I wondered if I could meet the challenge! Also, given the added burden of dealing with the fear based mentality of the early 1990's, I knew the trip was going to be very important for a whole lot of reasons! I needed to model my clarity and process for the others.

My fears were quickly dissolved, as Gerry became the "star" of the group. He is a very charismatic person with lots of dynamic behavior, and he was in his "best" form. I encouraged him to come forward with his process, as I believed that he had an important story to tell. He was accepted wherever we went. We all learned as we walked the path together. The next year when I was planning another trip back he said he wanted to go again. He had cashed in his life insurance policy to fund his trip and said, "If I am going to die, I might as well live it up!" Each year Gerry became stronger and clearer in his purpose and healing.

This next trip he took the instructor's training for HT. Through my encouragement he presented his work at the Holistic Nurses' Association of Australia. Everyone recognized the importance of his message and listened with keen interest. During this trip I became sick with a cold. The cold passed throughout our traveling group. I was worried for Gerry, but he did not get sick! I thought it was very significant someone with a very compromised immune system stayed well. The difference between him and the others, me included, is that he spent more time on self-care! He knew if he didn't, he would die!

Over the years I watched Gerry develop his expertise in Healing Touch as well as continue his service to his brothers and sisters living with HIV/AIDS. He spent many days and nights helping others on their path from what he learned along the way. He is a hero to me and I will never forget how the course of his life was changed with Healing Touch, and mine as well by walking the path with him. One of the most cherished moments for me was in 1998 when Gerry phoned me and said very excitedly, "I just had my regular battery of tests done and they can find no trace of the disease in my body!" I cried with him and walked on cloud nine for days. I prayed my thanks for Gerry, his journey, and what he was teaching us, knowing that he worked his way back to health from having nearly died several times. To fight back from a zero T-cell count and to not have a relapse since giving and receiving HT are things we need to understand. I give honor to the power of his spirit to return to health. I am grateful that Gerry is sharing his story, knowledge, and expertise as a healer. May we find ways to multiply this story and positive outcome for others.

Mary Jo Bulbrook
Carrboro, North Carolina

Living with AIDS

In 1992, I decided to change my health insurance and was required to be tested for HIV/AIDS. I was shocked when the test came back positive. My health remained good until the fall of '93 when I got pneumonia and thought I was going to die. I kept getting worse and saw my life in review. I remember how things smelled when I was in the 1st grade. My cells were not getting enough oxygen and it was like a pre-dying thing to me. Non of the drugs seem to work for me, until I finally got one that turned things around and I was released from the hospital.

In March, 1994 I had a relapse and it freaked me out mentally. I took it very hard and started seeing a psychologist. Going back and forth to the hospital was hard on me. I never looked bad as I was, but because I looked bad on paper I received Social Security disability.

My T-cells went down to eight. I was one of the lucky ones that had health insurance to cover my medical costs. This was due to the fact that in 1981 my mom insisted that I get health insurance. It paid for everything. I was able to get treatment that my friends and others were denied. This was my biggest non-personal factor of my recovery.

Two severe bouts with pneumonia were behind me and I struggled to maintain my health. Then Healing Touch opened a world of hope and healing within me. I went to a gay spirit vision conference where I met Gerry Mitchell who changed the course of his HIV/AIDS status with the help of Healing Touch. He worked on me using Healing Touch. It was so powerful and also changed the course of my life. It was like in the Wizard of OZ when Dorothy opened the door and everything became Technicolor!

When Gerry did a round of Magnetic Unruffling I could actually feel it become better on each side. Then while doing Chakra Connection his hands felt like they were emitting soft healing light. The immediate feeling and change lasted a couple of days. Gerry suggested that I take baths in Epsom salt and I followed up on his suggestion.

I was invited to go to a weekend for HIV impacted people but was not going to go at first. However, my colleagues at work encouraged me to go, so I went and took my friends with me. It was there that I met two HT instructors, Jane Hightower and Anne Boyd, who became my teachers in Healing Touch. They were wonderful!

I started taking Healing Touch but was not a particularly star pupil. I had to take Level One five times before I "got it." As my work in Healing Touch continued, I found that the energy I was modulating to clients was slowly changing underlying beliefs I held about my inability to be healed. This was also at a time when new drug combinations were sending my T-cell count back up. I was thus better able to accept my own healing and I am sure that affected my healing.

Healing Touch Level III is the practitioner level and it was a life-changing experience for me. In graduate school I had studied and then "forgotten" an Old Church Slavic text about a man who received a new heart by having the old one ripped out. During the course of the weekend this I found this happened to me.

I felt in the course of the five healing sessions that we were required to do, I was being totally rewired. I watched my old heart float out and a new one was put in. Driving back to Atlanta there was an opening in the sky that was beautiful. It seemed as if it symbolized what I was going through as I opened, the colors returned and life was beautiful again! I felt renewed and was a different person. That changed feeling stayed with me for several months.

Afterwards, to my puzzlement, it became difficult for me to work on clients and not take on their "stuff." I would be really exhausted after a session. I became curious, and with the pendulum began to check out my field. The first thing I noticed was that my field was full of holes! Each of the seven layers needed to be checked separately. For the first few months, a day would not go by when several layers needed to be "filled" again and again.

Then I became curious about the systems of my field. I began using the pendulum to check my endocrine, lymphatic and nervous systems. I checked factors related to HIV—T-cells, liver function. Thus I learned to keep tabs on my energy field. As long as I got plenty of rest, it was no problem to work on clients! And the more I worked on myself, the longer things held. It was a small but logical step to start asking the same questions about my clients' fields. I became more attentive to issues in separate layers. I checked organ function and system function, and made the interventions where appropriate.

Strange to say, the weaknesses in my field have forced me to become more aware as a Healing Touch practitioner and bring this knowledge forward. If I had not needed to do self-exploration to figure out what was going on with me, I would not have so quickly had to learn about the systems of the field and the more subtle qualities of the outer layers. I am grateful for the contributions Healing Touch has made in my life and am committed to help others on their path. Since taking HT, I have not had a relapse and my T-cell count is over 300!

Roger Weinstein
Atlanta, Georgia

Helping David Say Good-bye

I met David in 1991 when e came to my holistic nursing practice after learning of his HIV status. We reviewed his options and those factors that led to his disease, but little did either of us realize the real reason for our contact was helping David say good-bye.

Recently David lost his partner of ten years to AIDS. He had worked through a lot of his feelings about the dying experience with Frank and knew that he needed to get on with his life. Few knew about his status and his relationship with Frank. It was the early days when there was such a lack of understanding and acceptance of AIDS that the disease went underground yet influenced the entire world that didn't want to look at the implications of what was happening.

David was dreading fulfilling a promise he made to Frank before he died, that he would drive from North Carolina to California with Frank's car and take some of his other belongings back to his family. As David shared about his commitment to Frank, I saw a presence around him and felt it was Frank. The sense I got was that Frank was behind David and had his hand resting on his shoulder. I hesitated telling David about what I saw since I had not had the chance to share my background with David of being able to connect with Spirit. I did however suggest to him that whenever he felt too overwhelmed or upset that he should place his hand on his left shoulder. I could see that there was a presence there for him to tap into. We had planned to meet when he returned from the journey, which was to take two weeks.

On his return, I was met with a beaming client. When I asked how the trip went David exclaimed that it was one of the most meaningful trips of his life. What happened is that during the drive he kept thinking about his life with Frank— bring up memories and then letting them go. He had no idea that a flood of memories would surface. At times he would become overwhelmed he said, and he would then place his hand on his left shoulder as I had instructed. He said that a tremendous peace came over him and he felt the presence of his deceased partner. It brought tremendous comfort to him in his time of need! The trip turned out to be not so much to return Frank's belongings to California, but a way to provide David and Frank with remaining time to grieve, let go, and return to peace.

Mary Jo Bulbrook
Carrboro, North Carolina

Treating Kaposi Sarcoma: One Facet of AIDS

I met TJ at a "Learning about Healing Touch" workshop at the AIDS Survival Project in Atlanta. I was impressed with the attentiveness with which he was involved in his own healing. When I suggested he add Healing Touch to his wellness practice, he readily agreed. We decided to start with five sessions and then reevaluate. TJ is retired and lives with two cats. He had been involved in remodeling his apartment since 1991 and "has more gardens than Adam and Eve." He is currently doing volunteer work as an HIV+ peer counselor once a week and serves on planning committees for several HIV related organizations.

TJ is currently under the care of an OD, a chiropractor, and herbalist. He is taking a variety of medications for HIV including a protease inhibitor which is interfering with his liver's ability to process fats. He is also on medication to regulate his blood pressure. And since 1990 he has been under the care of a psychiatrist and is taking prescribed medication.

The first session's goal was to energetically balance him. During the assessment, TJ was mentally very alert, but not at ease. His body was rigid during the interview and he did not relax for quite a long time during the session. A visual assessment showed the left leg to be everted, whereas the right was stiff and vertical. A field assessment showed the seventh layer to be smooth and resilient. It was normal in every way except for a huge indentation at the right knee down the leg. The etheric layer was prickly throughout, especially over the liver. Intuitively I sensed that the culprit was the root chakra.

After doing the Spiral Meditation, TJ's body relaxed and a sense of peace and relaxation came over him. I followed with Chakra Connection to balance the field. Using Magnetic Unruffling I was able to remove particles of medication and tobacco in the field which resulted in clearing the field amazingly. The left leg was thick and gelatinous and the right leg was very dark and smoky. After about thirty minutes passed, the field finally cleared. The final assessment showed the indentation in the seventh layer to be completely gone. Afterwards, TJ reported feeling very relaxed and there was more color to his skin and he was not as tense. He reported feeling heat and pressure during the session. During the following month TJ had a recurrence of Kaposi Sarcoma (KS) which is an opportunistic illness that sometimes manifests in people with compromised immune systems. TJ received a round of chemotherapy to address the KS.

For the third session TJ was not very vibrant, as he was worried about the KS. He was to start a very toxic round of Interluken infusions soon but I sense a determination in him to do whatever necessary to maintain his health. In this session though the seventh layer of the filed was normal except for the fact that it pulled very close to his body toward his feet. He was still balanced from his self care as all the chakras were open. Hand scan showed that the etheric area over the spleen was very thick. I used Chelation to clear the system and Lymphatic Drain to boost the compromised immune systems. In additions since the back was blocked, I cleared it using the back techniques. After the treatment the field was full, field around the feet normal and the etheric layer even balancing out the physical aspect. TJ cancelled the next session as he was very ill due to the chemotherapy, however the KS had gone away.

For the last session the seventh layer of the field showed black energy on the edge above the head and a hole by the left foot. The entire edge radiated prickly static energy. The root chakra was open but the others were compromised probably due to the chemotherapy. I found problems in the heart energy as there was a black, snaking connection between the black energy above the head, and heavy energy above the heart in the fourth layer. I used the Spiral Meditation to open for deeper work, Full Body Connection to clear the energy and Magnetic Unruffling to address participate matter in the field from the medicine. It was extremely difficult to clear the field so I asked TJ to think of a steam iron to add steam to his first layer as I did the Unruffling. With this addition, the field cleared very quickly! I used Spiritual Surgery with light asking the guides to assist while modulating the complimentary colors of red and green. Although the black stuff didn't totally clear it was significantly reduced. I closed with sixth and seventh layer work and the spiral meditation. On final evaluation the seventh edge was free of black energy at the head and the hole by the left foot was gone. All static energy was gone and the right side was completely normal, whereas the left side was mush. The etheric layer was much better and less dense and less hot.

TJ reported after the session was that he felt 100% better. His gaze was more direct and several layers of static were gone. TJ had successfully fought off KS and made great strides in recovering from the chemotherapy used to treat KS. Healing Touch had helped his body maintain its best level of balance so that other treatments could have maximum effect and to minimize or reduce side effects of the treatments,. A wonderful addition to the treatment of KS!

Roger Weinstein
Atlanta, Georgia

Lessons and Insights:
1) The treatments used to deal with HIV/AIDS wrecks havoc with every aspect of the person's system. The side effects and subsequent assault on health is tremendous.
2) Any attempt to document what we are finding from those who are sensitive enough to pick up things is critical to the energetic management of this disease. Roger's descriptions are very visual and graphic what he is sensing and seeing in the field. His insight have helped me tremendously in showing what the effects are of chemotherapy. The aura pictures he has drawn are very helpful in understanding what a person is up against.
3) Another concept Roger and I have talked about in this work is the fact is an awareness of seeing the AIDS virus in the layers of the field. His question to me was, "If the virus is in the layers of the field etherically, should we not be able to remove it?" We have been successful with other conditions such are removing tobacco years after a person quits smoking and removing the effects of pollution and medications in the field! Why not energetically remove the etheric aspect of the AIDS virus and see what that does to the virus itself! Remove the feeder to the virus! A simple yet profound statement that needs to be researched This set me to thinking that as energy workers, we needed to band together and bring our intuitive gifts into play to see if we can get a clue how to treat AIDS/HIV energetically, a worthwhile challenge!

Offering Healing Touch with AIDS Patients

Last winter I was one of five HT practitioners who took part in a grant funded study at a nearby medical center that was designed by a HT colleague as part of her work in pursuit of a Ph.D. The study is in progress so this story reports a few of my experiences with permission of the principal investigator, Jo Wheeler Robbins. We were required to provide only the Chakra Connection in 20-30 minute time frame once a week for four weeks. While there may be protocols for different diseases that can be helpful and more specific, this study opened my awareness more to the power of intention regardless of technique used. Some of the reported responses from clients I worked with were:

Client 1 (after just one session—1 week past treatment): "I'm still the primary caregiver of my terminally ill mother. I still have AIDS, but some how my life does not seem quite as overwhelming. I'm coping better."

Client 2 (after two sessions): "I've been a social hermit for the last year because of severe diarrhea caused by drugs I have to take. I've often even missed my medical appointments because of it. After the first HT session, I had no diarrhea for three days. After the second treatment I actually went out with friends for an evening for the first time in a year. I feel like I have my life back."

Client 3 had significant neuropathy in lower extremities and was walking with a cane. He had a lot of leg pains. The feeling in his legs improved enough by the end of four sessions that he no longer needed to use his cane. He also related that his T-cell count had doubled and Viral load had dropped significantly during the four week treatment period as checked by his private physician.

The study ended after four months. It was a rewarding experience even if just for client feedback (official data from study not available yet). I also wanted to find a way to make HT services available to the clients in the study if they desired to continue.

It took a few months to get a clinic organized, but currently we hold a HT clinic twice a month that offers nine client appointment slots each clinic. The services are provided by Healing Touch students under the supervision of myself and Barbie Dunn, another CHTP. The HT clinic is held within an existing medical clinic that provides services to the Richmond Community. There is no charge to clients and it has become a vehicle for clients to receive HT, students to gain experience in working with clients with serious medical problems, and a way to provide a much needed community service that has increased awareness of what HT has to offer among the medical staff who work with this population. The client who was able to set aside his cane became an active volunteer in helping getting the clinic started and in ongoing support.

In the several months from when the study ended until clinic was opened he reported that his lab results had shifted from the gains he had made and he was again having a lot of trouble with his legs. Since he began receiving HT again he reports improvement in feeling sensation in his legs again and that he is able to go three days without a pain patch after each HT treatment. We are continuing to keep records and track what seems to help and how often HT is required to maintain decreased or relief of various symptoms. It seems from this experience that HT is a valuable supportive therapy for clients who are dealing with HIV as expressed by direct client feedback.

Deny Brown
Richmond, Virginia

Midwife to the Dying

Hello Fellow Healers,

Namaste! As a Healing Touch practitioner living with AIDS, I have worked with hundreds of clients with HIV or living with AIDS over the years. I find the potential of sharing our experience in this forum and in a larger context very exciting. My particular calling is as midwife to the dying. I have found many ways to employ an eclectic combination of Healing Touch, Reiki, and massage to this community of sacred brothers and sisters actively looking at death. I especially look forward to hearing and sharing all the variations of the Chakra Spread that have been used with clients. It certainly remains a tremendously powerful tool in my practice.

I have been with many at transition and just a month ago lost another very dear friend to AIDS. At some point I look forward to writing and sharing the larger story of how energy work supported my friend Bruce as well as his family and the broader community in a beautiful piece of forgiveness and letting go.

The corner stone of the work is in creating the sacred space where clients are more able to connect with spirit and hear their guidance spoken in their hearts as they make personal choices in the process. I also have created a Sacred Seven Circuit Labyrinth floor cloth for this purpose.

In one month's time, I am hoping to participate in the 1999 Parliament of the World's Religions in Cape Town, South Africa. I will be joining my spiritual teacher and guru M. Jaya Sati Bhagavati in bringing the AIDS Quilt to Africa for the first time. I say "hoping" as part of my on going challenge is creating the financial prosperity to support this work. There is a great deal of leg work involved in walking this path, but each of you are blessings along the journey.

Feeding the soul with Love and Light,

Gerry "Dancing Dolphin Durga Das" Mitchell
Atlanta, Georgia

Healing Touch Partnerships HIV/AIDS Team

For years I have had a premonition that I was going to be working with AIDS population. However, over the years I have had limited occasion to do so. Nothing matched the original feeling I had until now.

In my Healing Touch Level IIIB class in 1999, Roger came into my classroom. As I listened to his experiences and heard about his work, I sensed that he and I were to do some work together. He described some wonderful experiences and the depth of his clairvoyant ability exceeded the norm but it came across like a wild horse that needed some guidance!

We began to share experiences together. I sensed that his insights were extraordinary and would give us clues as to what was going on in the energy system of those struggling with HIV/AIDS. As Roger proposed questions to me, a flood of insights came while were speaking. I decided then and there, it was important for me to move forward now and connect people I knew throughout the world to begin tackling HIV/AIDS energetically.

My intent was to link energetically those who had expertise of different kinds to pull our abilities together and see if we could get insight as a team of energy workers tackling the disease process. I invited people to join the effort after explaining the purpose. There was much excitement generated. I knew this was the start of some very important experiences.

While counseling over the phone last year with a client who reported feeling low in energy, I could see a hole in his energy field and gap between the fourth and fifth levels in the energy system. I advised him to come for a treatment to patch up what I was seeing. I also got the message that something that happened several years ago was related to this tired feeling. I was trying to find an association. As we continued to talk the client reported he recently met someone that created intense feelings in him. This new person reminded him of a old relationship where he felt like there still were things to work out! We began to explore the relationship between the recent symptom and the unresolved emotional issues. This experience taught me about the importance of understanding the interrelationship between all aspects of our being: physical, emotional, mental, and spiritual.

This experience and others reinforced the importance of meticulous data collection to look for pattern from those we work with that will offer new insights on how to intervene. I have witnessed the tremendous clinical progress that has been made as we did this. To this end, the newly formed HIV/AIDS team has linked their gifts of various kinds to collect data and begin to test out some new possibilities in energy interventions that may be of assistance. The research reported briefly by Deny Brown offers some sense of direction and insight as to the potential impact on this disease. It reminds me what history has taught us in regards to medical advances based on astute observations that let to breakthroughs in health care. I believe that linked together, energy workers can do the same, especially as they link closely with Spirit to be led beyond the human into the Divine. Hence, this is the purpose of the team! Some of the insights from this pioneering work will be reported in later editions of this book and through other means as well.

Mary Jo Bulbrook
Carrboro, North Carolina

A Clairvoyant's View on AIDS

(Editorial Note: Following is a reading done by a nurse and medical intuitive on the AIDS virus. Nancy is a Healing Touch Practitioner and is a participant in the HT Partnerships, HIV/AIDS team. The goal of the group is to poll our intuitive gifts and see if we can evolve a worldview regarding the identification of the AIDS virus as it comes to those with Higher Sense Perception. Each of us makes intuitive contributions. We then condense the data to lead to energetic way to manage the disease process with the state of knowledge we have at this point in time. Then we will move to develop clinical studies so the scientist can verify what has emerged. This is very exciting pioneering work and is by no means a finished product. It is reported here and now to stimulate you thinking so that you can share your process with the team as each of us has a piece to the puzzle. We need the clients, their family and friends, and health care professionals to be open to receive and flow with what comes. With Nancy's permission I have edited it to create, "A nest for the information for us to examine and process further." You will know what is my input by the italics as I built on the foundation Nancy Stonack presented.)

The following intuitive reading is a presentation of an energetic profile of someone with the AIDS virus. The goal is to understand the energetic profile that could then serve to point to a sense of direction for the energetic interventions. I started to read each chakra, read the symbols of them, and soon realized that I was presented with was a worldly universal contract to have this disease. In other words, those who have the disease have accepted the burden for the world to heal pain that is multigenerational and multidimensional which is why the current paradigms are limited to eliminate the disease. What is possible however is to be able to heal as one accepts the dimensions of multidimensionality and created treatment strategies that keep this principle in mind. The virus seems to flourish when it is kept one step ahead and seemingly out of reach.

In other words, when dealt with as in the future or the past it seems to grow. The more grounded the better. What actually dissipated the virus was bringing the virus into present time. As I dated the virus to the current date, it could not exist. When an individual is always in the future and trying to find ways of catching up with a cure, our energy is in the future and not in the present. When the individuals energy is fully in the now and in the present, the virus had difficulty sustaining its' vibration.

I was never quite sure if the virus came first and then the damage to the chakras or if the damage was there and then came the virus. I now however know it is the damage first.

The first chakra was brown in color, and very damaged. It was clear that the individual came into this lifetime with it already blocked from past life times. There were lifetimes of processing death, and grief. The virus thrives on the dead energy and the first and second has no life force energy in it at all. There is a lack of self-nurturing ability where the person came into this life never being able to connect with one who wanted to nurture. The old contracts seem to be housed in the first and second chakras. The individual carries the contract through several lifetimes. The individual has done this contract for so long that they no longer remember another way. There is need for big time work on outdated contracts and past lives is a key and bring all of the information into the present. Then the virus cannot exist as far as I can tell. The second chakra was a very black, and held grief and loss of past lives. They came in with social and emotional emptiness.

The third layer was yellow, a powerful yellow indicating the power of the virus was within the energetic system. But the chakra was still not spinning as it was stuffing too much in, taking on too much (being accommodating, trying and making everything fit and work). It just never stops, but keeps going in a survival mode. In this layer was the dollar sign. It is tied into giving too much value to material things. The disease is there, to teach lessons around inner focus not outer focus and to value the individual more that material items in life.

The heart chakra was black and white with a green underneath. And victim and martyr stuff around grief and death and devastation. The fifth layer completely was separating the first, second, third, and fourth from the sixth and seventh. There was a black band that went all the way through the throat area. There was complete separation of the body and the spirit in communication abilities. Removing this black band would assist the individual in regaining part of their ability to have some spiritual perspective. The virus survives on the divide and conquer theme.

Part of the contract of coming into this life time was to process the grief of many lifetimes for many people. (This means to me that those who are suffering are suffering for us. They have taken on the burdens of many who have been hurt as the residual pain of many generations has coalesced so to speak, into this other reality to finally be healed. It is as if society figures out a way to cure, heal or prevent certain disasters and then something else comes along and we are continually challenged to clear from before.)

Contract came up in the sixth as a scroll. We are people who understand the meaning of life. We are born to communicate about death, grief, sorrow, fear, sadness, and change. We are about devastation. We are not without purpose. We understand and know the sorrow that feeds on us. Others in society help us to rebirth sorrow into a new light. For it is this new light that will rebirth us all. We are honored to be here. We are honored to be doing our world. We honor all those who share the processing of pain.

The seventh layer had Supreme Being energy as it was Godlike energy, silvery type with radiance. The Genetic Code is set up on this layer. Part of the contract is to work on this as a spiritually challenging test. Contracts, again, that the individual agreed to before coming into this planet. Letting go of control and the mechanic of life. It is about letting go on a very deep level. A huge group has agreed to move to a similar destination. The same Rhythm, same pace, for the overwhelming devastation in our history. Helping to make the planet and vibration healthier and to help with the process of the grief left behind. The spirits are very powerful to be able to take on such a contract.

Part of the intervention is to teach people with HIV/AIDS different ways to process grief. Can they process of enormous amounts of grief without having to die? The upper body shifted to the right and the lower is shifted to the left. Balancing past life work and teaching techniques to process grief.

Cath Webber-Martin in Australia also describes a case in point related to what Nancy is talking about in this book. Her article is titled, "Healing the Present, Releasing the Past."

In closing I am reminding the reader that what Nancy and I are suggesting is to take this information into your process in working with HIV/AIDS. Let us know what you discover around this as we attempt to bring together intuitive data to help provide with a sense of direction beyond where the efforts of medical scientist are looking. When we come up with clear strategies and we are getting some clues as indicated by some of the work reported here, we will then be in a position to add this dimension to the research efforts of scientists.

Nancy Stonack   Mary Jo Bulbrook
Tacoma, Washington   Carrboro, North Carolina

Needing To Let Go
"Tell him he needs to go on so he can be free." These were the words that came to me for one of the participants during a session while teaching an Energetic Healing workshop titled, Healing Wounds in New York, February, 1999.

Each workshop in the Energetic Healing program begins with a meditation and process to access areas that need to be worked on by the participants. Therefore, in addition to the educational goal of learning Energetic Healing, each participant is guided through personal work that is initiated during the opening meditation lead by the instructor.

The meditation sets the stage by accessing unconscious material that has influenced the energy system of a person both in and out of awareness. The process is influenced by calling in Spiritual Guidance for not only the individuals, but the group and instructor as well. Therefore what happens in a session is determined by many factors: issues/needs of students/participants, the "group" effect of being in relationship and in community, and Spiritual direction that is accessed.

At the end of the workshop when we were completing the last intervention, the student healer asked me to help her with her client who was having excruciating pain radiating down her arm that she did not have when she came into class. As I walked over to help I was thinking, "This is not the ordinary way to end a workshop." I wonder what we are all going to be taught by this.

As I approached Helen, the first things she said to me, "Remember I was the one you gave a guided message that said, 'Tell him he needs to go on so he can be free.'" I asked if she knew who it was. She said, "Yes." She thought it was her husband who died nine years ago. Helen also reported that during the meditation she had a "sense of a energy mass" in her field. It was dark in her imagination. "I had the pain in my right arm like this several weeks ago but not when I came to the workshop. I need to get rid of this pain as I can't stand it!"

I called over Jean Gustafson, who was in instructor's training for Energetic Healing in this class, to work with me as it is important to prepare new teachers how to handle the "extraordinary." I then turned the classroom over to two other instructors in training, while Jean and I focused on Helen. If I did not have help in the classroom, the work would need to be referred to another time and perhaps require bringing in other health care professionals, not unlike what the medical profession does in providing traditional health care.

I told Helen that I needed to ask for guidance to identify what might be most helpful for her. Jean and I separately in different parts of the room centered, went inside to get clear, and asked for guidance. After a few minutes I approached Jean and asked what guidance came to her. She said, "We aren't done yet. I can't leave until we resolve the issues about the kids. You are still so angry."

I thought it this was interesting because something also came to me about kids, but I thought surely it does not have to do with the kids! How easily we can ignore what comes to us when the first insight can be right on!

As Jean shared with Helen what came to her, she gasped and said, "My husband did something to one of the children and I am still very angry with him and couldn't forgive him. He died suddenly without my being able to say good-bye and deal with our unresolved issues."

Even though I am a therapist, I knew since this was a classroom experience in energy work it was not appropriate to do psychotherapy, as my role was to give and teach energy-based care. Therefore I said to Helen, "Take time to deal with your unresolved issues with him and call me over when you are finished." Jean and I went to sit down and hold the light for her to do the work.

After about ten minutes Helen called us over and said she was finished. I then told her the additional information I got when I prayed, "What do you want her to know?" I was told, "I'm sorry, it was time to go. Don't be afraid. I stayed behind to support you. I have been afraid to let go and go to the other side. I know it's time to go. I want to take you with me!"

I said to her, "Do you want to go?" Helen quickly replied, "No! I want to be free and let go too."

Helen described that four years ago she had the identical pain she experienced in the workshop. She had tests done and was diagnosed with breast cancer and had a mastectomy. It is as if the pain returned to the other side of her body and was continuing to give her the message to finally work through the issue of unresolved anger in order to "Let Go."

I said that it appeared as if he was pulling her with him by the arm, affecting heart chakra as a result of unforgiving anger that eventually led to breast cancer. I repeated the message that came to me and asked her if she wanted to go with him. Once again she emphatically said, "No!" I said, "It is now time to release him."

I gathered the energy up in my hand using Unruffling while she focused on releasing him. I then Lasered the energy connection and strings attached to her, scooping him up to the light while calling for someone to come and meet him. The process took only about five minutes. The pain left and she was very overwhelmed at what had just happened. She reported her experience to the class.

Mary Jo Bulbrook
Carrboro, North Carolina

Lessons and Insights:
1) Unresolved anger holds people and issues to us.
2) A person cannot go to the other side without being forgiven. I do not know if this is true in all instances.
3) There are energy ties that bind us together in this life and in other time dimensions.
4) The spirit world is interactive with the physical world only we need to know how to interact with it.
5) Jean who never had interacted or "talked" to spirits like that before was able to pick up the message from the deceased man that was the key to her healing.
6) This work can be taught to those who never think they could do it.

7) Physical manifestations are linked to real life dynamics in a person's life and needs to be dealt with as well as the physical manifestation—maybe even more so.

8) The progress of the soul is shaped by our life experiences both in and out of consciousness.

9) We are multidimensional beings, simultaneously interacting with other realities.

10) Energy work can go deeper and quicker to resolve psychological dynamics that are held in place by a "event" and "time" energy "file," so to speak.

11) To heal, one needs to change the energy dynamics of issues either in or out of awareness.

12) Spiritual Guidance is the most important resource a healer has. Learning how to link with ones guides and help the client to more fully access his/her Spiritual base is one of the highest callings of a healer.

Circle of Healing

During the closing moments of our IIIB last day's morning meditation, I had a striking vision. I felt a pull to open my hands energetically as if reaching for the hand of the person on either side of me. I experienced a clasping of hands proceeding around our circle. When the last energetic link connected, the joined hands of light rose into the etheric vehicle of the earth's aura, and separating, reached out a hand to all healers and light workers around the globe. Hands of light called forth other hands, offering love and support. I saw connection touching it in joy, love, and compassion—reaching out to create a link, one hand touching another. With each new link, the hands rose higher and higher until they began to fill the entire auric field of our planet. As hand upon hand filled the space, the hands of the Blessed Ones of Light-Love-Wisdom, and all the helping angels and guides added their hands over the multitude of hands filling the field. It was a promise and a blessing of love and hope and united purpose.

Barbara Rulf
Springfield, Virginia

5 | CONNECTING WITH ANIMALS & LAND

Healing To and From Animals

My New Animal Spirits

Having to make the decision to put my beloved pets to sleep was very painful on many levels. This is not unlike what others have had to go through. When I returned home in March, 1999 from my trip to New Zealand I was not prepared for the intensity of the demands on me. After a short while Ginger, my beloved pet of 17 years became desperately ill which demanded me to care for her that took about four hours a day. The care included the following: lifting her to go outside to the bathroom, standing her up to go for a walk, feeding her tenderly and searching for anything she would eat, cleaning up accidents throughout my office and upstairs in her favorite spots, taking her on trips to the animal hospital, and giving her healing treatments.

The demand was great physically and emotionally. She however got through it! Only to then be confronted with Chaney, her mate of 17 years, having a fall that left him in discomfort. So once again I went into action doing all I know to do. My "animal expert" friends in energy work kept talking to me about letting go. Although I thought I was ready, are we ever really ready? Chaney fooled us all as well and once again pulled through.

I had planned a family holiday in Hawaii to celebrate my children's graduation from college. After settling into our home away from home, I received a call from home that one of the dogs had been rushed to the hospital. I couldn't believe it since they were both well before I left!

When I called the animal hospital I was surprised to find that Chaney was paralyzed. The doctor said he may have a brain tumor or a stroke. Chaney was resting comfortably and would be looked after by the hospital staff, but he asked what I wanted to do? I couldn't believe the stress on all of us in Hawaii and back home. How could this have happened. I wasn't ready.

Donna had stayed behind to teach a workshop and would be joining the family gathering after the weekend. I asked her to go the hospital and give me her opinion what we needed to do. The weekend was filled with anguish as I tried to sort out my feelings and determine what was right.

On Sunday night after visiting Chaney in the hospital, Donna suggested that she take Chaney to our vet and get his opinion. She went home exhausted after teaching, the stress of the situation, and the drive home from her workshop three hours away. Donna prayed for a sign from Chaney what needed to be done.

Upon arriving home she went inside and tipped toe to see Ginger from the top of the stair as there was not a sound coming from the room. She then went to bed exhausted only to be awakened by the thrashing of Ginger downstairs 30 minutes later. She rushed to Ginger's side to find a very distressed dog with liquid pouring from her ear and blackened liquid all over the office downstairs. She scooped up Ginger and raced her back to the hospital where Chaney was. They admitted Ginger in critical condition.

Donna called me with the sad news. Now there were two decisions to make. We knew it was time and that this was the sign from Chaney. They needed the family to be gone so that they both could be released from our love and make the journey for their transition. The next day, Donna drove the two dogs to the vet at another hospital. He agreed to come to our home and put the dog to sleep.

Donna came home with both dogs and spent the entire day preparing them for their transition. She took them to their favorite spots in the yard, carried them around the lake behind our home, let Chaney chase a duck saying, "If you can get him Chaney, you can have him," knowing all along that Chaney could not catch the duck. Chasing the ducks was one of his favorite pastimes. She sat on the bank behind our home talking to them telling them we all loved them. She also prepared their grave site with the help of a friend.

Meanwhile, back in Hawaii, each family member prepared to let go. We were together as a family and said our good-bye's and worked on settling our intense emotions. When your children grow up with the animals, it is a lifetime of letting go.

The time had come. The vet came to the home. As each beloved dog was held and gently talked to and released from his/her physical body the tears began to flow as the physical life energy left their bodies.

Chris who had lovingly cared for the dogs over the many times we were not home, heard Chaney speak to her. The vet as well heard Chaney speak. Donna said that she had never witnessed such love and caring from a vet and our friends. She was honored that we could create such a loving way to say good-bye.

In Hawaii as I said my good-byes and with tears flowing I called home to hear that the transition had just taken place as I dialed. The energy connection between my beloved animals and me was just as connected then as before. Their passing marked a transition for our family that is very significant. After the event I can look back on what happened and be at peace. What happened next completed the process for me.

My family left to go home to NC after a week, while I stayed behind to teach a workshop on Energetic Healing under the able coordination of my friend Lori Protzman.

During the workshop I was sitting on a small raised stage so that I could watch the group do the healing. We were in a church setting. I had in my lap the EH Notebook that I was correcting. I was preparing for the revisions of the book and doing it during the workshop helped me to remember what was important that needed to be changed.

Suddenly I was compelled to stop what I was doing and just sit and look over the room. I felt very peaceful and content, but kept wondering why I was not writing and what had come over me!

Suddenly Lori Protzman sat up and looked straight at me, started to cry and motioned for me to come over. She had been on the table receiving a healing. When I approached her she could hardly speak.

Between sobs she said that during the healing her cat who recently passed away, Ku'u, had come to her. I had been in communication regarding her beloved pet. Lori had been the one to track me down on holiday to tell me that they were trying to reach me regarding Chaney and Ginger, so Lori was very familiar with what happened to me.

She said, "After I was petting my Ku'u's spirit, I was told to sit up. When I did, I saw you directly in front of me on the stage area. There were two dogs with you, one on your lap asleep and one under your chair resting comfortably." When she described them, I knew they were Ginger and Chaney coming to be with me, comfort me, and help me in my healing work. I will never forget the peace I experienced at that moment, and know what is available to each of us as we learn to connect with guidance, including animal spirits!

Mary Jo Bulbrook
Carrboro, North Carolina

Animals Owning Healership

I have been blessed with the presence of animals throughout my life. However, it has been only since I initiated the Healing Touch for Animals / Komitor Method of Healing program that the recognition of the animal healers came to my awareness.

A sense of awe comes over me as each four-legged friend enters my workshops, hand in leash, with their two-legged counterparts. Not only were the people coming to learn to work with the animals, the animals too, entered the class to learn this work. I have seen transformation of the animals during these times. The animals may not understand the words spoken or the ideas of the teaching, but they understand the energy as they experience the techniques. They then transfer that energy experience into an inner knowing to step into and own their Healership.

One of my favorite stories is about a golden retriever named Fancy. She seemed invisibly haughty as she sat through the workshop. Her small body-frame, light-buff color and shy presence made her seem fragile as she stuck close to her person, Ellen. Fancy's training, however, awarded her as a certified therapy dog and she worked with people in the nursing home. She also participated in obedience trial competitions, but her greatness was hidden by the invisibility she held. Ellen, out of frustration, was in the workshop to help Fancy with her low self-esteem and the stress induced colitis she would experience during competitions.

During the workshop, Fancy would allow others to practice the techniques on her during the hands-on exercises, but she became uncomfortable whenever Ellen left her side. As I supervised the practice sessions, I was reminded of Fancy's presence. Throughout the day a gentle, "Oh, and there is Fancy," would come to my awareness, as if she were peeking out from behind a door. She did not cower or hide, but it seemed as if she would disappear and reappear at will.

The interesting thing was, Fancy held such greatness when she allowed us to "see" her. Her energetic being was like a queen, stately-dressed in velvet and ready to attend to very important affairs. A specialness of this elegant creature would let itself be known and yet the specialness would be confused by the invisibility. As I left the workshop, reflecting on the animal participants, I again remembered Fancy's gentle beauty and then all thoughts of her disappeared.

Several weeks later, however, I awoke from an uneasy dream, with confusion running through my head. Fancy, this dog who left my thoughts so easily only weeks before, had come to me in the dream. She was speaking in words I could not understand. I heard a human voice coming from this dog-being and could only decipher an echoing babble. As I moved through my day, thoughts of her and the dream would continue to nag until I called Ellen. Sharing my dream, I asked if I could do a long-distance healing session with Fancy. I felt very strongly that Fancy needed to tell me something. The uneasiness continued to bother me and I wanted to release the dream.

As Fancy's session unfolded, she needed to be anchored into the greatness that I had sensed during the workshop. The balancing, clearing and strengthening of her energy field came easy because of Ellen's routine energy work with Fancy. Fancy was ready to embrace who she was. During the session I could see and feel her come into an understanding of her purpose. She was ready and able to take on the role of healer, leader, and teacher. The babble ceased and words were no longer necessary. Fancy's clear and balanced energy settled in silence.

Ellen reported Fancy's colitis stopped. In the weeks to come, Ellen began to see an unfolding as Fancy adopted her new essence. She was sure of herself and no longer became nervous at the competitions.

Fancy also took on the role of healer. She stuck by the side of another family dog through his dying process, comforting him, and easing his pain. This healer dog then consoled Ellen and her husband with their grief. Several months later, a new puppy came into the household. Fancy began to train the unruly youngster in the ways of a dog. With gentle discipline, she eased the integration of his energetic and pesky presence into their family unit.

Did Fancy come to the workshop just because Ellen insisted? You be the judge. I feel she came to the workshop seeking help and to embrace the healer that she was destined to be.

I have seen many of my animal students transform. The work easily changes the way they function in relation to their people and other animals. Understanding their purpose and the energetic components of the healing work, the animals embrace and own their healership.

Carol Komitor
Highlands Ranch, Colorado

Messages from our Winged Friends

Last night I opened randomly one of my books, not unlike I usually do to ask for Spiritual guidance. I turned to page 95 in *Animal-Speak: The Spiritual and Magical Powers of Creatures Great and Small* by Ted Andrews. At first I said no, this must not be the page I am to read, as it is not one of the descriptions of the animals. I paused and reminded myself to read the page and see what it had to teach me I knew I needed to follow guidance and not intellect..

The section spoke on the mystery of feathers and flight. As I began to read, I then knew why I needed to read it, as it has a story to tell! The work describes the important role feathers play not only for flight, but also for every "kind" of flight. Little did I realize then the full implications of the description. Andrews states, "Every kind of flight requires a unique wing construction." He explained that the bone structure of a wing is like a human arm structure except in the hand section. The fingers of a bird are fused and longer to help with flight. It is the hand of the bird! "Different birds have different styles of flight," he reports, and consequently they need different wings structures. As you examine the bird totems, he says, "See what kind of flight it will help you with in your life."

Andrews says that there are different kinds of wings: some for maximum lift and ability to soar and glide (big, long and broad wings), some for great speed and ability to maneuver (small, swept-back wings), some for reflecting lots of energy to flap and easy ability to glide (long, narrow wings) and some designed for great power with fast take off (short, broad and arched wings.). Each type of wing has its own meaning and purpose.

The two most dangerous moments are the taking off and landings. This signifies movement into new dimensions in ones life. This is not unlike what we need: balance, and control, learning to leave the body and re-enter takes preparation. The animal's guidance is needed to tell how to achieve things in life: Do you need outside sources to give you a lift? Also what helps you to land on your feet and be secure from that flight? What makes you feel safe and guided? Do you have the right wing span?

My life has been guided and assisted a lot by winged animals. Here are some of those stories. I have collected feathers most of my adult life for some unknown reason. In my travels throughout the world I usually have a communication from some bird about something. Below are several communications through the mediums of feathers.

Mary Jo Bulbrook
Carrboro, North Carolina

Holding Hands with Karl

I can't believe he killed himself. Enraged with the news given to me while attending the American Holistic Nurses' Association meeting I sought to find comfort with having to deal with the suicide of a young gifted man from Australia. Karl was only 19 years old when he took his life. I had only met him briefly a year before, but he changed my life through our connection.

Karl was an old soul in a young body that was dealt a hard life this time around. He had been making progress with his extensive gifts as a healer but did not have enough grounding to hold him to this plane. Looking back there were signs of his impending choice but they did not change his destiny. He had tried several times before but pulled himself through. This time he accomplished his goal.

I was in uncontrollable anguish at the news. I was leaving USA in three weeks to join Karl in Australia to help him launch his work and teachings and accompany me with my work to help others heal. Thoughts went through my mind: "Could I have said something different to alter the course? Did he need something from me I did not give or could not hear? What was the meaning?"

As I walked from one building to another in complete shock, I asked for a sign from him that he was on the other side and OK. Just then I walked into a building and found a feather inside the building on the path. I picked up the feather, held it to my heart and felt close to him, as he knew I love birds.

I left for Australia as planned. When I arrived at the home where Karl had lived for almost a year with one of my best friends, everywhere I turned there were memories of him. My friends insisted that I work through my grief. They made me travel with them to the place where I had last gone with him the year before. Karl had driven me to Nimbin, a small "hippy" town about one hour from Lismore, New South Wales. On the way he had pointed to a very sacred Aborigine men's place and had told me about the story related to that site. As we drove past the site I was reminded of the story and the time we stopped there and got out of the car to look at it.

My friends said, "It is time to get over it, try to communicate with him on the other side." I said, "It is not like holding his hand. It was not the same as I had many conversations with spirits and that is not what I wanted!" My friends listened patiently as I ignored their request.

On our trip back from Nimbin we approached the site that was very sacred to the Aborigines and important to Karl. In the middle of the road was a beautiful bright colored bird that had just been killed on the center of the road. We had not seen it before. We stopped to remove it from the road so that no one would run over it. As we got out of the car and gently moved the bird to the other side, my friend driving the car asked me if I would like some feathers. She also asked me if I would like to take the wings. I said yes as it is important to bring honor to the animal and I would be sure to keep the spirit of the bird in memory as I have many feathers from my travels over the years.

We buried the rest of the animal in ceremony and quietly made our way back to the car. In silence, we drove home. Shortly I felt intense heat come from the feather and my awareness shifted to the wing. I felt the energy surrounding my hand. It brought me great comfort. I then realized that Karl was holding my hand. Earlier I had said, "It is not the same not holding his hand." So from the other side, once again, I was moved into another dimension of communication as the "hand" of the bird held my "hand" through the spirit of Karl. Birds are our messengers if we learn to read their messages. Today that wing has a place of honor in my healing space.

Mary Jo Bulbrook
Carrboro, North Carolina

Ducks are Birds Too

The passing of Rosie was a New Year's Day I will not forget. Early morning on New Year's Day I did my usual morning ritual of feeding the ducks on the pond behind my house. As I threw the cracked corn out the ducks came up hurriedly quacking in their usual noisy way. I lowered the corn to the eagerly awaiting ducks and then saw them go back to the pond. While watching them return to the pond, I noticed one of the ducks swimming by himself, very isolated and I sensed something was wrong. Sure enough, I found the duck had something wrapped around his neck. I became angry as I thought, those kids were at it again. This time they have left the duck with something around his neck. Don't they know that it is wrong to hurt animals like that.

I tried without much luck to get the end of the string. The duck kept moving out of reach. Finally I was able to corner him and pull him to shore. Much to my dismay I realized he had a hook swallowed down his neck. I carried the frightened duck up the hill to get help in caring for him. I called for my friend Donna to come and help me remove the hook. We tried for about an hour with no luck. We then left the house together to go to the vet for help wondering who we might find open on this holiday. The first vet looked at us and I could tell she did not feel secure in helping us. She worked for about another hour with no luck and sent us to another emergency hospital. The same pattern was repeated—more attempts and no luck.

This current doctor said that we need to take him to a bird specialist! "A bird specialist?" I said, "He is a duck!" Needless to say it was the first time I realized ducks were birds. I know at some level I knew that, but I only thought of them as ducks!

While waiting to be seen, I looked into the eyes of the duck and experienced being touched to the depths of my soul. I started Unruffling him and to my amazement the duck's energy released and filled the room with an intense comforting energy. I had never experienced anything quite like that in healing individuals. The experience of the energy was in waves and expanded intensely throughout the room. I knew that the duck had a healing and I did as well.

So we were off to find the specialist to help retrieve the buried hook. When I brought the duck to Dr. B he asked me what the duck's name was. I said he is just duck! He was not a pet but just one of the ducks in our neighborhood pond that I feed. Dr. B said that he would not work on the animal until he had a name. So the duck became Rosie.

Dr. B worked for several hours once again without success. He returned and said that he needed to operate and did I give him permission to do so. By this time I couldn't even imagine how much money we had spent treating the animal that wasn't even ours on a holiday to boot. But I was too far into this by this time and consented.

We left to get something to eat while Rosie was being operated on. Coming back from the restaurant we both had a bad feeling that things were not going well. The doctor met us at the door with a guarded report. Rosie had swallowed the hook and it did more damage that he anticipated. If Rosie made it she may have more problems and did he have our permission to put her to sleep if he thought her quality of life was compromised. We agreed and left with heavy hearts.

At the end of a New Year's day that was spent in three animal hospitals we received a phone call from Dr. B that Rosie needed to be put to sleep and he was sorry. His gentle reporting of the event and caring was so wonderful that Dr. B taught me wonderful principles to keep in mind! All things have an identity and are not just "ducks." I was taught patience, giving and receiving love. I had communicated to the depth of the soul with this animal and in return, Rosie had shown me the other reality of consciousness of ducks!

Oh yes, I forgot to mention, none of the doctors charged me for caring for Rosie. It was their gift to us for caring for Rosie. What comes around, goes around!

Mary Jo Bulbrook
Carrboro, North Carolina

Visit from the Duck Spirits

There was a pair of ducks that hung out in my front yard under the bird feeder waiting for some scraps to fall. Often I would say to them when I walked out the door, "This is not a good place to hang out. Chaney our dog would love to have one of you for lunch." But my pleas when ignored. One of the ducks was limping and in discomfort and the other was her loyal mate. At times when the other male ducks found her they would aggravate her to mate with them. More than once I rescued her from their unwanted advances.

This day when I came home one of the ducks was missing, not the one injured but her mate. I began to worry and went searching. Several days later I found him killed by some animal on the side of the pond. I worried about who would protect her now that her mate was gone. So I became a duck guardian. I knew that was not a good role for me since I travel so much. I penned the duck up underneath the porch so that no other animals could get to her. Finally I called the animal control to take her to be cared for as she was grieving and did not look well.

After I made my decision, I left the makeshift little pond (an over turned car luggage carrier) where I had bathed the duck and worked with her to help her heal her leg. After several conversations with Carol Komitor (Healing Touch for Animals), I sensed it was time to let go. I went back to the office and began to work as I waited for the duck to be picked up.

Finally I decided I could not stand it any longer. I walked to the protective place I had my little friend and sat in a chair to tell her good-bye. I heard a human voice from the duck tell me he appreciated my caring for his mate. He had come back for her and would take her to the other side.

"A duck is talking to me?" I wondered. I thought I had gone mad, but sat there calmly. Then the mate came to me and sat under my arm as if I had my arm around him. Together we sat in silence as we both looked at her and released her from the physical plane. When this was finished, the duck from underneath my arm came directly in front of my eyes and pecked me on the forehead. I heard a voice that said I was being marked for all time so that ducks everywhere would know I was a friend to ducks!

I came into the house wondering what I had just experienced! I may be making this all up, but then all of my life is just making it up. Everything I have reported happened. Animals can speak, if we learn to listen and how to listen. They have emotions and feelings, and need to be loved too. The care and love I gave these specific animals I also sent as a pattern to the soul group of birds and have told them I will continue to champion their cause to communicate to humans. They have a lot to teach us if we take the time to listen and understand.

Mary Jo Bulbrook
Carrboro, North Carolina

Duck, Duck, Goose

Tonight Jim and I went to a barbecue at Lake Wheeler Park in NC. It was given by the Wake County Meals On Wheels Program. It was a lot of fun. Good company, good food, a live band, and a beautiful natural environment. After we ate we walked down to the lake and the water was beautiful with the glittering setting sun. The music from the boathouse was "Pachebel's Canon" As we sat on the bench at the water's edge some kids were feeding bread to about 30 ducks and geese. After the bread was gone the kids tired and walked away. The ducks and geese were milling about, some in the water and some on the sand. I looked at them with the intention that "If there are any of you in need of healing come to me." Immediately one came walking toward me followed by another. They walked right up to me paused for a moment and walked off to the side to nibble on the grass. Still within my aura. One lone duck then walked straight to me. As he walked I noticed that he was "pigeon-toed" and with each step he stepped on his on feet. He was in pain. He stood in front of me for almost three to four minutes. He turned and looked me straight in the eye for a long time. We were Present for each other. Awesome! Being in the right place at the right time healing happens.

(Later I looked up Duck in the book *Animal Speak* and it said: "Because of its connection to water, it is linked to the feminine energies, the astral plane, and to the emotional state of humans. Ducks can remind us to drink of the waters of life as well as to nurture our own emotional natures.")

Cathy Mack
Garner, North Carolina

Blessings from a Sparrow

I dropped Ted off for his radiation treatment, parked, and went back toward the hospital to be with him. Just in front of the hospital entrance I saw a little sparrow lying still on her side, eye blinking, but with barely any chest movement. Two sparrows flew down to check on her, paused to take a look, then flew away. I withdrew a tissue from my handbag, carefully scooped up the sweet little critter, and began Unruffling. I walked back and forth, Unruffling and asked the assistance of the devic kingdom for the sparrow's highest good. After about five minutes the bird moved her head looking around. Then in a beautiful burst, she flew out of my hand up into a nearby tree. What a beautiful blessing to fill my heart that had been heavy that day.

Barbara Rulf
Springfield, Virginia

Angel Work

I came to Healing Touch through my own process of healing and self-care. Healing Touch and Energetic Healing helped me so much in my own health journey that I began to use it with my animals and others who came to me. I call what I do, "Angel Work."

Since I have learned Healing Touch, I have had many opportunities to use it. In addition to the regular sessions with clients, I use it in creative ways that I am led to do. I first began working on my animals. (I have three cats, two dogs, three goats, one horse and six horses that belong to my boarders.) Whenever any of them seem a little off I check them out and send healing energy. Two of my animals have epilepsy and require daily mind clearing to control seizures. I do this at any time and any place or wherever I happen to be. For I believe if they come into mind, they need something from me or I need something from them. So I just send healing light and receive it back!

I branched out into working on friends or acquaintances that needed a boost of some kind. For example, doing mind clearing when someone was upset or doing an Energy Drain and Replenishment from the Energetic Healing Program on a harried friend. When I wake up in the middle of the night and can't sleep, I'll tune into who needs work and lay in bed and work on either a person or animal asking that their highest good be done for the healing. Not my will, but thy will. I find myself being asked by the universe to work on various people and or animals that I don't even know. My life has become a constant prayer of healing, giving and receiving, receiving and giving. I have helped many others and they don't even know consciously that someone has been sending absent healing! For this reason I call what I do, my angel work, since angels often work behind the scenes to help us when we are in need and forget to ask. I love doing healing work and it has kept me well!

Eileen Gress
Apex, North Carolina

My Dog Ben

I have used HT with a number of animals, some of my favorite creatures on earth. One was my dog, Ben. He had skin irritations especially during the flea season. Considering the fact that he often slept with me, this became an irritant to both of us. One of my favorite techniques with him was the Magnetic Unruffle. He would be scratching and scratching when it was time to sleep. So I began doing the MU at these times and he would settle down in minutes. Usually it took very few passes to calm him and the longer I did this with him the more he and I both benefited from it.

Carol Kinney
San Anselmo, California

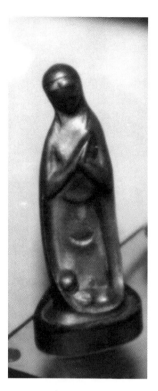

Share God's truth by your beingness. Take each moment of the day to be your prayer, your offering to make this world a better place, for in doing so the 'whole' will be changed. Peace starts at home - in your heart, in your being - with those you love and those who are hard to love. Once this truth is realized this age will be transformed into a new golden age with less pain and suffering. Service is the tool to salvation of the self and the world. Align your will, life, love with God's.

Rainbow Image of Mary
Clearwater, Florida

www.marytalks.com

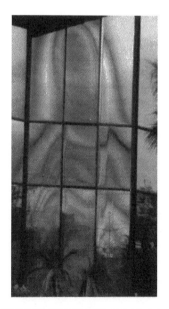

CONNECTIONS WITH MOTHER MARY

JOURNEY TO THE LIGHT

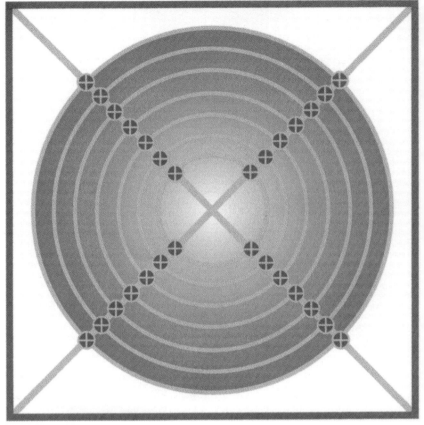

Energetic Healing through the Pyramid Labyrinth

Focus on the four directions and archangels (Uriel, East-Emotion, Gabriel, South - Physical, Raphael, West - Mind, Michael, North - Spirit), seven chakras or seven layers of the field.

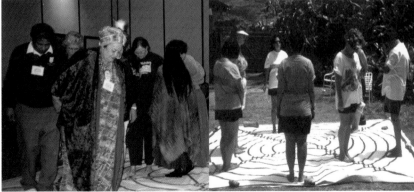

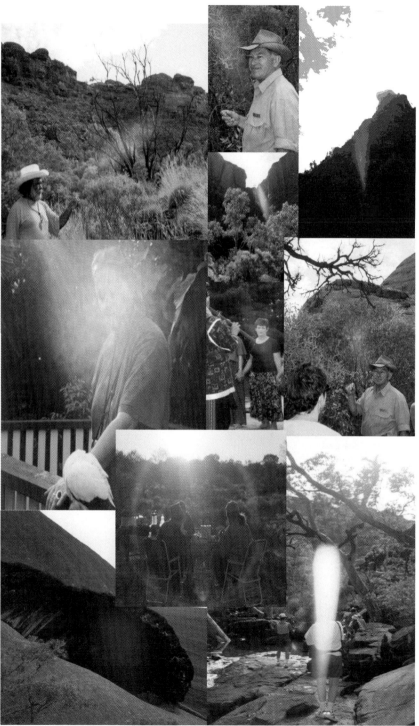

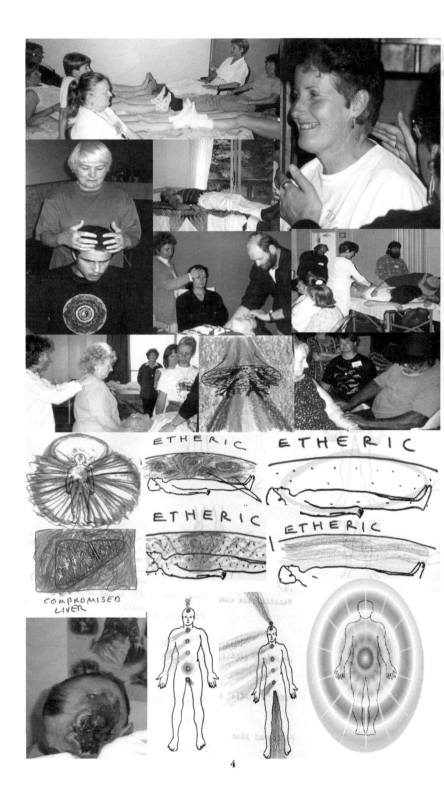

ETHERIC

ETHERIC

ETHERIC

ETHERIC

COMPROMISED
LIVER

4

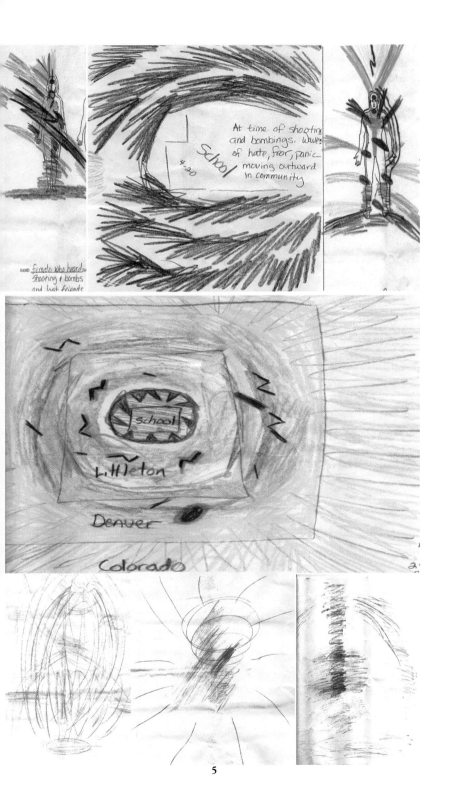

At time of shooting
and bombings. Waves
of hate, fear, panic
moving outward
in community

School
4-20

NAME female who heard
shooting + bombs
and lost friends

school

Littleton

Denver

Colorado

5

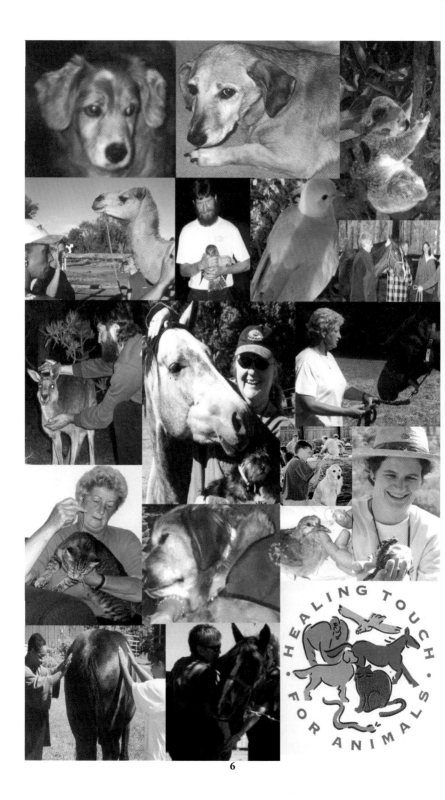

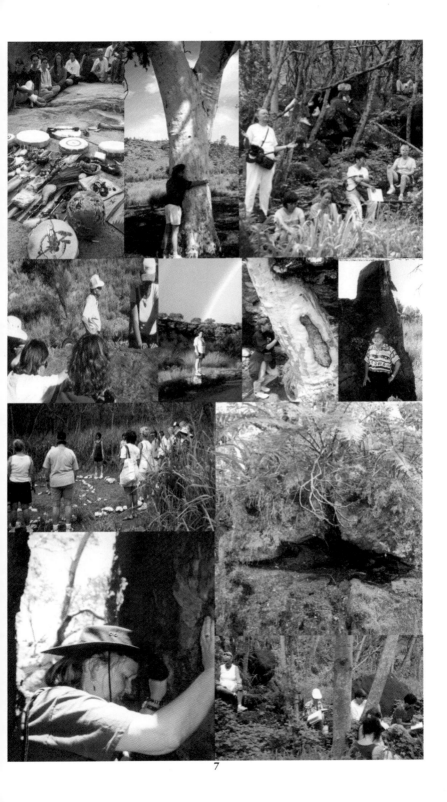

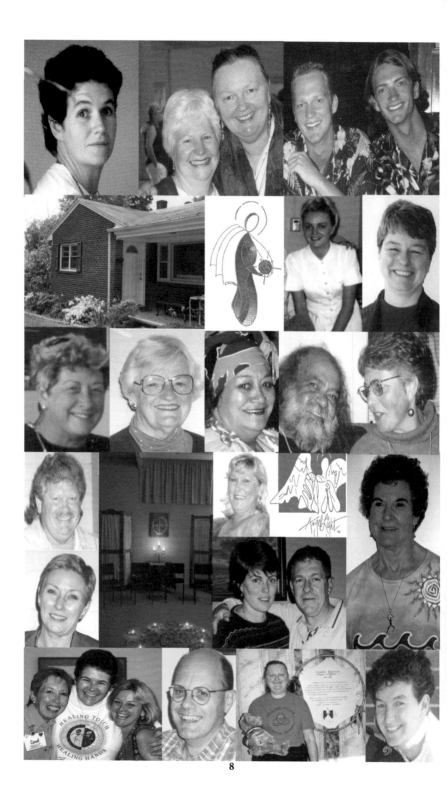

8

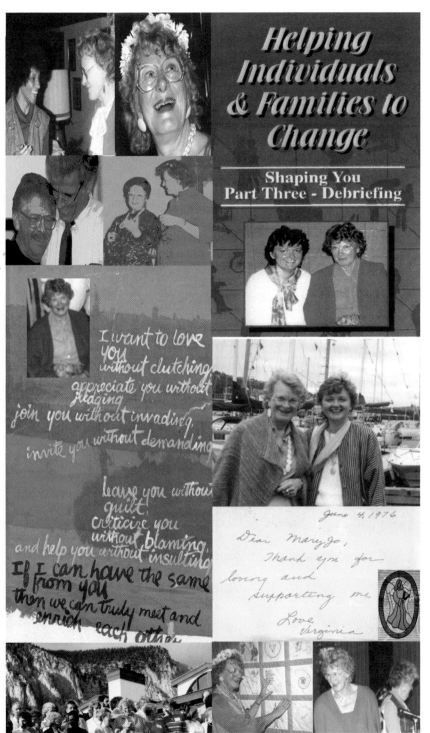

Helping Individuals & Families to Change

Shaping You
Part Three - Debriefing

I want to love you
without clutching
appreciate you without
judging
join you without invading,
invite you without demanding

leave you without
guilt,
criticize you
without blaming,
and help you without insulting,
If I can have the same
from you
then we can truly meet and
enrich each other

June 4, 1976

Dear Mary Jo,
Thank you for
loving and
supporting me
Love
Virginia

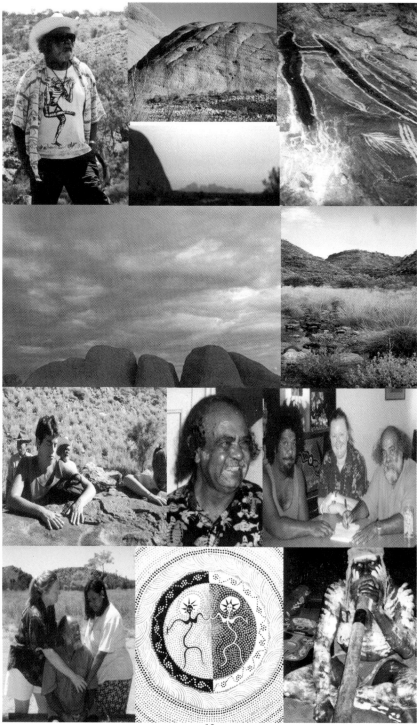

10

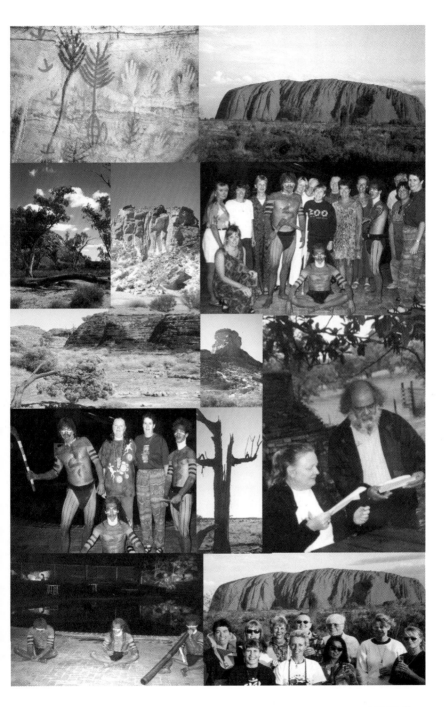

ABORIGINE / HEALING TOUCH PARTNERSHIPS

11

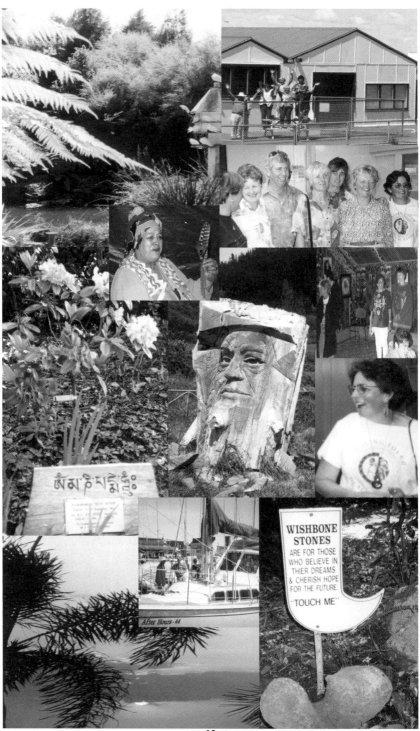

WISHBONE
STONES
ARE FOR THOSE
WHO BELIEVE IN
THIER DREAMS
& CHERISH HOPE
FOR THE FUTURE.
"TOUCH ME"

After Hours 44

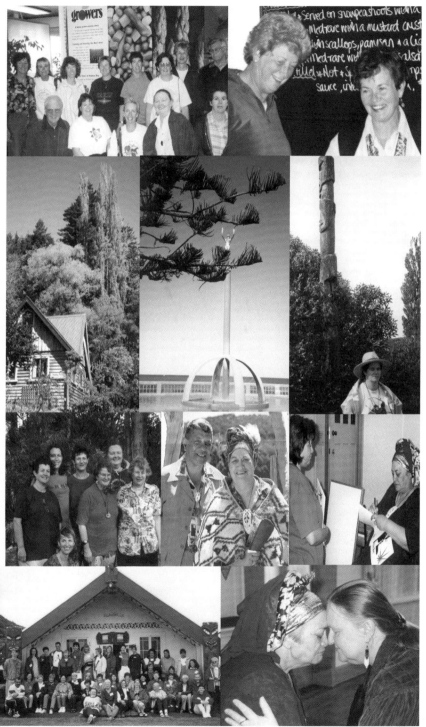

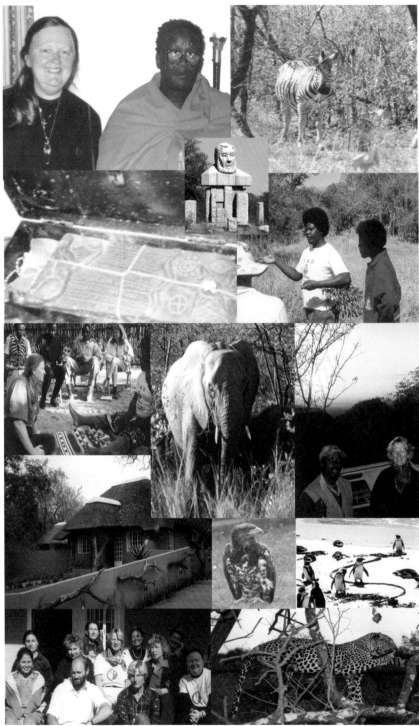

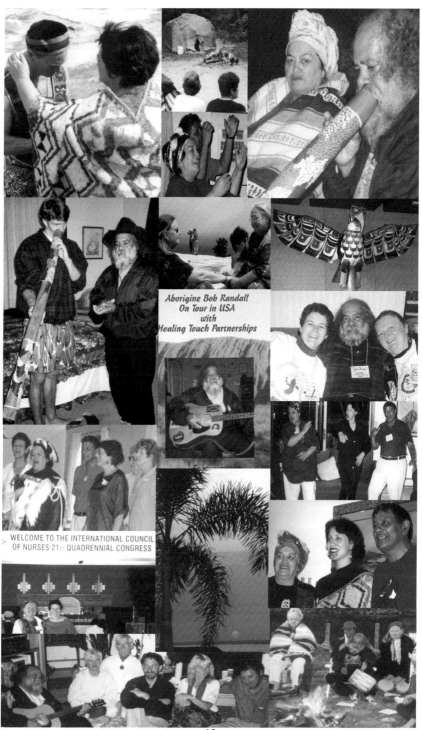

Aborigine Bob Randall
On Tour in USA
with
Healing Touch Partnerships

WELCOME TO THE INTERNATIONAL COUNCIL
OF NURSES 21st QUADRENNIAL CONGRESS

15

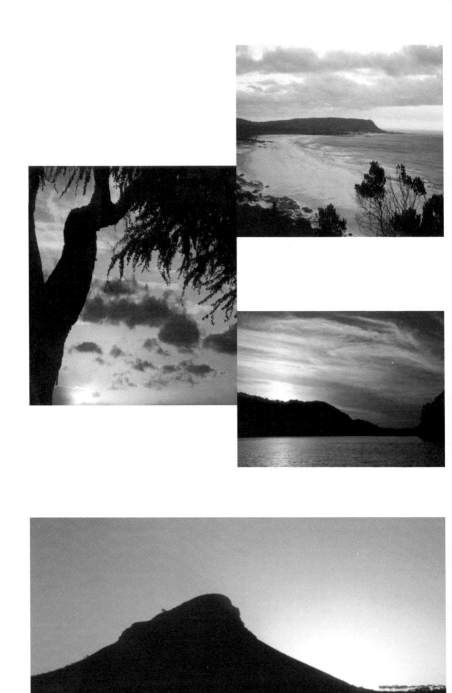

Messenger Pets

I was trading energy sessions with another CHTP whose name is Barb. I asked her what she'd like to focus on for that session. She responded that she would like to reach some clarity about where the energy work was going to fit in her life. She stated that her shiatsu practice was growing, but her energy based practice was pretty stagnant. She felt she needed to take her work somewhere, but she didn't know where. Barb got on the table, and we set our intent that Barb would receive some information during this session to direct her on her path. Barb had some flute music playing in the background. I asked her if she minded if I changed the music. She said it was okay, so I put on Richard Shulman's *Assissi*. This album is very spiritual as it was recorded from Richard's experience visiting the sites of St. Francis of Assissi, a special friend to animals. I worked on Barb for some time. I did several techniques primarily from the Energetic Healing Program, namely, Inner Core Balance to connect the self inside energetically followed by a Seven Layer Drain and Replenish which takes out the old and replenished with healing energy.

My next technique, was the Hara Alignment to connect one with one's life path and highest purpose. As I began the technique, Barb's animals came into the treatment room. The big, black lab kept bumping and licking me. The cat, Ms. Purr, kept moving under my hands. This was strange behavior for these animals. Typically, they remained quiet until our sessions were finished. I continued the technique. As I made the final connection between the Soul Seat (point connecting the self or innermost desire) and the ID point (identity of the self), Ms. Purr hit my hand and bumped Barb. Barb opened her eyes briefly, then closed them. I finished the session with the Chakra Blessing. After the treatment, Barb stated she had her answer. Healing Touch and energy work with animals is her life's path! Spirit told her through Ms. Purr, Shadow (the dog), assisted by my choice of music. Spirit gave her not one, but three cues, as to the direction her healing work. Needless to say, Barb listened and is now involved in energy work with animals.

Jean Gustafson
Scotia, New York

Lessons and Insights:
1) Pay attention to everything that goes on during a healing session, and sometimes before and after too. Often times there are important clues from Spirit that you need to learn.
2) Animals are teachers too. Learn to listen to them.
3) Focus your healing to solve problems and receive guidance for specific requests.
4) The right music will enhance a healing.

Bosley's Adventures

My friend Susan, has a 5 lb., 9 year old Pomaraniam dog. They have a special bond, but Bosley has one actively that frightens them both. On a number of occasions, Bosley has disappeared, always returning, but in his own time. Susan tells me one time Bosley actually went a distance of 30 miles to return home alone through the highway system in the Los Angles area. Bosley is black and is trimmed like a very small bear. Recently when Susan and her husband Brad were constructing a fence to assure Bosley remain closer to home he disappeared again. This time he was gone for four days and everyone was called to send love and safe energy to him and support all efforts towards his safe return. I got involved with Bosley too and actually had a dream that he would return.

On the fourth day a neighbor called and he had been found on a construction site. He apparently was trapped in that location and was heard as he cried for help. We were all relieved and again puzzled with his adventure. Why did this little being decide to go off again on his own? Didn't he see the danger? Apparently not! Training to be a better communicator with animals, I decided to ask Bosley what this was about and to explain the stress it caused for all concerned. He replied simply, that he likes being free to explore and adventure on his own. He remembers being both a mountain lion and a horse in other lives and flashed me a picture of a huge Black Stallion with rippling muscles. He said he simply forgets how small he is now. We discussed how scary this is for all concerned and he has not left since.

Carol Kinney
San Anselmo, California

Helping Buddy

I was able to follow through on your recommendations Mary Jo to help Buddy by using Inner Core Balance on the etheric and fifth levels of the energy system, that you teach in Clearing the Internal Self. Buddy is 14 years old and is fading in health. He is so much a part of our family and I hate to see him suffering so and a times feel so helpless. I was delighted that he relaxed and was able to move his legs more easily after the treatment. He slept on his side instead of guarding with the back feet tucked under (which I think injures them more). He is much calmer and more playful now. So, thanks for the suggestion. I hadn't thought of doing EH on the animals, but I will from now on!

Carol Wander
Woodenville, Washington

Australian Animal Encounters

Not too many people get to give healing on Kangaroos and owls! While I was visiting my friends Paul and Sandy Forman and their children at their home in outback Australia, we shared many wonderful experiences. Some of those experiences were with their animal friends. Their home, built by Paul and Sandy, is a marvel and story in itself. Needless to say, the magic one experiences there is wonderful.

Paul has a thriving Healing Touch and massage practice that provides home care and love to the people of his town. If you can imagine a one street town having a booming energy-based healing with massage business in bush country, well, this is it. I wouldn't have believed it had I not experienced it myself. Needless to say, Paul and Sandy's home is a haven for those in need, including our animal friends.

Can you imagine, healing a kangaroo? I was there on one such occasion as verified by the picture of Paul working on one of the many animal visitors to his property. This picture is in the HT Partnerships brochure that describes our new program titled, "Natural Health for Animals."

There she was, just as bold as anything, coming for her afternoon healing. Paul tells stories of his many encounters over the years. Some come for play, care, and comfort. One such story was receiving help to die. Imagine, animals coming for help to die.

Another occasion that was magical was a healing on an owl that had been hit on the road. We were leaving late at night about 10:30 p.m. on the way to where I was staying, when Paul suddenly slammed on his breaks. He said, "I saw an animal on the side of the road and think he has been injured." We both ran from the car and standing there was an owl in all of it's beauty. Being so close to all these wonderful animals awed me.

Paul gently picked him up and held him tenderly. I crawled behind the car seat and we drove a block down the road to an eccentric woman who cared for animals. Her yard was literally filled with "trash." Paul stated that she was a wonderful loving person to the animal kingdom but being neat and tidy was not her specialty!

When we pulled into the driveway I saw he was right. A hesitant woman came out to see who was pulling in late at night. Paul explained what happened as she gently took the owl from his hand. When he did so, the owl looked like someone had turned out the lights as his energy dropped tremendously and he began to fade fast.

Immediately I placed my hands over him without thinking or hesitation and started Unruffling him. The woman exclaimed in surprise, "I can feel that." Only five minutes passed and the owl opened his eyes, perked up and I knew he was through the immediate crisis.

I will never forget my encounters with the owl and kangaroos of Australia. The feel of their energies is not like any other. Their quick response is wonderful. I am pleased to have energy first aid available at all times. In energy work, your tools are your hands and heart with Spirit ever guiding, ready to spring in action when needed!

Mary Jo Bulbrook   *Paul Forman*
Carrboro, North Carolina   *Anakie, Victoria, Australia*

Horse Connection: Rebuilding Energetic Bonds

I was called to see a friend of mine who had experienced her second fall from a horse within a very short period of time. When I was finished healing work with her I asked, "What about Spider?"

She said, "He is out in the paddock." I said that was not what I meant, but I guessed that Spider had not seen her since the accident, and that was four days previously. "Is that correct?" I asked. "Yes," she replied, as she had not been able to get outside.

Previously he had seen her twice a day for feeding. He had seen her taken away to hospital, been brought home by someone else, and then not seen her since. I wanted to know what this had done to his energy field. I went out, caught him, took his cover off and talked to him for a while before assessing his field. I found that he had completely blocked/closed down his mental field. A technique to deal with this was not immediately clear. As I drove home I received the information I required.

The next morning I returned and took the owner out into the paddock and sat her on a chair holding the very end of the lead rope. I then proceeded to drain the horse's mental field both sides. I then asked her to create a positive happy picture of herself interacting with Spider and to hold this until I asked her to stop. It is very hard work for most people to maintain a concentrated focus. She had to hold it for nearly 15 minutes while I refilled the field with love and calm. I then let him go. He walked backwards and forwards to the water trough not sure whether to drink or not. This is a normal reaction after this level of energy work. He came back to his owner and rested his head near her chest. This was the reaction I wanted, that he be firmly linked with her. I was just the facilitator.

His owner reports that there seems to be a much closer rapport with Spider than ever before. It is my belief that traumas need to be thought about in their broadest sense and rectified as soon as possible. I am looking for these throughout the field and am now rectifying if possible with the assistance of the owners. This is long overdue work. I am working with their spiritual fields as well. I shall report more at later date as their spirituality stems from a different highly evolved being and works in a slightly different way.

Annis Parker
Christchurch, New Zealand

The Animals Call to South Africa

As I was preparing to go to South Africa I had several unexpected animal visitors. Jenna Vos and I were traveling together and had put in a request to meet with some native healers. Jenna is a South African who lives in Byron Bay, New South Wales in Australia. She is a HT Practitioner and HT Instructor. It was through her contacts that I first went to South Africa.

Jenna had been given two free passes to visit a Wild Animal Game Reserve due to the fact Jenna is also a travel agent for her brother who runs a luxury train (Rovos Rail) through the country. One of my loves is connecting with animals so I was looking forward to visiting the Game Reserve. We had scheduled two days to visit Ulusaba, a Game Reserve located in the Sabi Sabi Sands Private Reserve adjoining the Kruger National Park.

One of the women in Cape Town where I also planned to teach HT wanted me to come early to Cape Town and for television and radio interviews. Going there would mean that I had to either not go to the Game Reserve or leave early. At first I said yes that I was willing to go, but on second thought realized that I really wanted to see and interact with the animals. I postponed a decision however to get guidance as to what I needed to do.

During the night, a vision of an elephant awakened me. It was as if he looked directly at me and into the depth of my being. After he left, a Zebra who did the same thing visited me. I did not know what these visits meant, but I took them as a sign that I was to not postpone or cut short my trip. So I informed a very disappointed coordinator whom kept begging me to change my mind.

When I got to South Africa, I began to understand the meaning of the visits. I met Credo Mutwa, a beloved Zulu healer, told him the story of my animal visitations the night before. Credo is a seer, sage, sangoma, inyanga, healer, psychic and storyteller—one of the most remarkable healers of our time. He has written a book describing the significance of the African animals. It is titled *Isilwane – the Animal: Tales and Fables of Africa.*

Credo informed me that the elephant was one of the sacred animals of South Africa. When I told him about the Zebra's visit, he said that was even more important because the Zebra signifies the black and whites coming together. Since that is my goal and philosophy, as I received assurance from Credo I settled down with my decision and knew I make the right one.

When I arrived at the Game Reserve the tour guides who met us at the airport and for the trip to Ulusaba exclaimed that he had rarely seen so many animals that could be seen from the road while driving through the National Park to the Resort. I took it for granted that must be the norm as I was greeted my almost all the major species of South Africa! It was only later that I realized the importance of this meeting of the animals coming to greet me.

The manager was glad to see us and exclaimed that the elephants had come to the water hole about stones through from our African first class huts that we were gifted to stay in. Within a short time of our arrival the elephants came back. This was an amazing sight. While watching close at hand in their native country, I was struck with the majesty of these animals and grew to have a great respect for them. I felt called by them to their country after my dream and the assurance by Credo that this was no little sign.

The Game Reserve we were staying in was quite wonderful—a "things to do" that would be an outstanding event in ones lifetime. The particular place that we were staying had several major negative events happen. It was touch and go that we would be able to stay there, as there was a fire that burned down one of the major lodges. Also, the week before we arrived there was another fire that almost burned the place we were to stay! The fire came within about 100 feet from burning our hut. The staff said that something was wrong. That comment matched what Jenna said before we left for South Africa when we were having difficult making arrangements to go to Ulusaba because of the mishaps. She said, "I wonder why we are being called there, maybe to help with healing." I was destined to go the Ulusaba.

As the staff talked about the problems an old woman appeared to me. I knew she had something to do with what was happening there. I told them and forgot about the old adage, "What will people think?" and just spoke my truth.

I was asked if I would go to the place where it burned down and see if something came to me. I said I would be happy to before we went out for our morning viewing of the animals. We were awakened at 5:30 a.m. for the trip up the large hill. On the top of the hill was a burned building and lodge. I saw the same woman who appeared to me at base camp. Her words were, "You no longer care about and for me. Until you change there will continue to be mishaps." What I was told by our guide, who was a native from there, was that place she was referring to was a sacred site that once overlooked a burial ground. The native people use to conduct ceremonies to the ancestors and have rituals to honor the dead. They no longer performed these rituals.

I told our guide, who was "called" to be a Sangoma (native African healer) and whose mother refused for him to have the training because it would mean he would be taken away from her, that he now had the information that could stop the tragedies. It was up to him to work with his people and return to honoring the ancestors and the ancient ceremonies. I had fulfilled my destiny and role and would await the next part of my calling.

Mary Jo Bulbrook
Carrboro, North Carolina

Meditation for the Animals
In the wake of Hurricane Floyd, healing is needed in many ways in North Carolina. During a group meditation I received guidance on working with animals. To care for the animals, we are to send healing energy to the group soul of the species of specific animals. The group soul of the dog, group soul of the cat, group soul of the horse, etc. The animals that are in the midst of the flood area are being spoken to by all the other animals. They offer them encouragement and love to endure whatever it is that has come to them. They are in touch with each other. Just as we humans are continuing to evolve, so too are the animals. This is part of their lessons. We are pulling them along with us to a higher vibration. The microbes in the soil down to the earthworms are all in flux. The vibrations of the Web tweak us all.

Cathy Mack
Garner, North Carolina

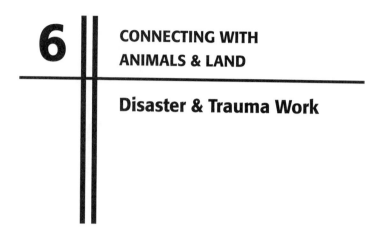

6 | CONNECTING WITH ANIMALS & LAND

Disaster & Trauma Work

Beginning Energy-Based Disaster Work

My introduction to the importance of energy-based disaster work started with the Cincinnati, Ohio Tornado that hit during the time that I was having an Energetic Healing Faculty meeting in Carrboro, NC. There were five people in the group whose lives were directly connected to Cincinnati including myself since that is my birth city. When I walked into the class on Saturday morning, I was met with a very distressed group. Some of them had talked to family and friends back home to get information about the impact of the disaster. The first reports that we received were that the office where one of the people worked was leveled and the tornado had touched down several times in the area. The extent of the damage was unknown.

The first part of a crisis like this is the impact of lack of information combined with the fear and overwhelming stress that results in an inability to concentrate on anything else other than the unknown. It is as if there is free flowing anxiety. The first process in this case is to talk and give everyone the chance to say whatever he or she needs to say. The second, following closely, is prayer. Asking for protection, guidance, and relief is very important. So that is what our group did. We talked about what we knew and what we did not know to determine what could be done immediately and what might be done in the next stages. The seeds for disaster relief work were sown then. I said to the group, "I wished there was a way to respond to the disaster energetically and I wonder if there was something needed by the community that energy workers could provide." Since this is uncharted territory, we were just groping our way in the dark. The process I outlined above helped us deal in our own way with the immediate crisis that affected us. To repeat:

1) Talk. We talked and brought up the energy and response to what was happening.

2) Pray. We determined what we could do immediately was to pray and focus the light to those in need.

3) Focus. We asked for help to focus our energies to shift repeated assault from other tornados touching down.

4) Meditate. We meditated to create inner peace surrounding intense worry.

The strategy worked. We were able to proceed with our agenda for the day and be productive, although off schedule regarding what was planned. I marveled at the capacity of human beings to work through things energetically. Little did the group realize at the time, I was functioning not just as a leader that day of training, but I was also actively working to deal with a collapsed class energetically. My goal for the day was to heal the wounded.

Mary Duennes took up the challenge to lead the HT/EH group into this uncharted area after she got home. A group of us committed to support her through e-mail (which has a rapid turnover of communication) as the events unfolded over the next couple of days and into the months that followed. Our goal was to focus, pray to God and our Spiritual Guides to get a of sense of direction about what we were learning as this experience was lived.

I called upon my skills in occupational health, crisis management, and psychiatric mental health nursing as well as an expertise in energy-based therapy. I became acutely aware of the importance of what we were attempting to do—to build a body of knowledge from a lived experience, create a valid method of research, collect data, process the information, and come forward with findings. Thus, we set out to launch a new field, Energy-Based Disaster Care.

Mary gives an excellent account of her team's process later in this chapter. As we were just getting settled from that crisis, then came the Littleton, Colorado crisis. The same group of people who were now committed to study the phenomena of disasters, natural and man made, focused our attention on the new disaster. What we saw and learned from that is reported by Janna Moll as supported by a team of HT/EH practitioners.

Then came hurricane Floyd in North Carolina, then a call from Texas for help with flooding, and soon the scope of the need for this field quickly became apparent. We knew so little and were not prepared. Anyone knows that in disaster planning there are drills of all kinds to get people prepared. Here we were, a large population of energy workers located where the world had its attention and we were unprepared! It was then I made a personal decision that I would focus my attention on this emerging field.

The questions that became apparent as we began our work in designing Energy-Based Disaster Care were the following :

- What are the dynamics surrounding the crisis and tragedies that need our response?

- How can the HT/EH communities respond?

- What is found energetically in the people, land, and animals?

- What worked to deal with the findings?

- What are the greater implications for energy workers world-wide to assist in management of disasters?

In an e-mail dated April 21, 1999 I outlined the charge to build a role for energy workers in response to tragedies including natural ones and those man made. I said in the note, "It was time to move beyond the individual to the broader social issues that are affecting the world in massive disasters from earthquakes, flooding, hurricanes, shootings, pollution, tornado and life threatening illness and plane crashes. Hardly a week goes by without some difficulty."

Some of the issues that need to be addressed in developing energy-based response and treatment protocols for disaster care include the following:

- Dealing with anger and rage that is stored and needs expression.
- Irrational outbursts to dispel the stored negative energy needing release.
- Massive destruction of lives, property and the land.
- Acute physical, emotional, mental and spiritual health needs.
- Spiritual crisis.
- Acute grief.
- Post traumatic stress syndrome.
- Long term grief.

Here are some practical, "working" solutions to address the emotional and mental needs of trauma and disaster relief in field:

From HT use Magnetic Unruffling (clearing field), Mind Clearing (stress relief), and Therapeutic Touch (stabilize the energy system).

From EH use Hara Alignment, expansion of the Core Star first (rebuild energy system), Energy Field Drain and Replenishment second (clearing), and Inner Core Balance third (reconstruct the internal structure).

Teach them meditation to balance the energy system.

Those who are intuitive, focus attention on the area and see what you get. Collect the data and see where it takes us!

I am suggesting that we conduct field research titled, Coping With Natural Disasters: Healing Shattered Energy in Peoples Lives and the Land—The Experience and Learning.

I anticipate the work will have these dimensions:

Clients: basic medical emergency care; short term emotional crisis; long term emotional management; clearing and physical stabilization of the energy field; preparation for flashbacks; grief work; dealing with shattered psyches; and finding meaning.

Caregivers: telling the stories; releasing the traumas; finding meaning; overwork and fatigue; emotional overwhelm.

Land: repairing unstable energy conditions as well as unstable physical conditions; sealing holes; releasing traumas; releasing trapped spirits; cleaning-up energetically as well as physically; rebuilding; calling back the plant divas; giving attention to the healing needs of all the animal species.

There also needs to be follow up on an interval basis as the impact hits different people at different times. Put a treatment hotline in place. Hold clinics on a regular basis. Focus on the needs of all concerned including the caretakers.

Some of the energetic things that we received I would like to report here. I have found it very useful to begin a collective effort to pool our intuitive gifts to get different parts of the puzzle intuitively: Regarding Cincinnati, I saw a hole, an energy vortex left in the land where the tornado touched down. It needed to be sealed to return the energies to normal and begin the healing of the land. There was also a broken line of energy around the main street that feeds into a larger mass. Cathy Mack's visioning is also included her story. The findings from Janna Moll and her group are also reported in the photographs section. Studying them and continuing this process will give us invaluable data for now and the future. Regarding the Littleton crisis, I saw dots all over the area, and Annis Parker from NZ got that there was sadness trapped in the atmosphere.

If we follow the concept that we are all connected worldwide, it becomes even more apparent how important to develop a constant vigil on this and begin to map the territory!

Mary Jo Bulbrook
Carrboro, North Carolina

Calling for Light and Love
(The following story is taken from two e-mails I sent to friends and colleagues in the Healing Touch community regarding the impending effects of Hurricane Floyd)

Date: Tuesday, September 21, 1999
Dear Friends,

Thank you for helping us divert the hurricane heading to our home and minimizing the effects of the storm. I dreamed two nights before I knew there was a storm coming that my home was shattered into pieces. I became very scared and did not know what this meant, so I knew that I needed to pray for healing.

I was teaching EH in Christina Lake, in Canada and called on the help of those attending the class. We did a meditation of protection for our homes and radiated that protection out throughout the storm's path. In addition we focused energy to assist those who had already been effected by the storm as well as the many lives and property damage that had taken its toll. After the meditation a woman reported seeing a hand come and lift the storm. I went to bed with a heavy heart, yet knew that we had done what was needed to get prepared. After talking to my family back home, who I joined with in prayer, I went to sleep.

I was awakened at 1:00 a.m. Pacific Time (PST) and had a visualization of a very large hand from the sky scooping up the what was in its path. (I had not remembered the information from the person in the mediation the night before.) Then I heard glass shattering. I felt though all was OK and I drifted back to sleep.

I was awakened again at 4:00 a.m. (PST). This time I saw pearls and white crosses with flowers. I became agitated and focused on my children. I intuited that they were OK. I then took out the pendulum to assess what had happened and it showed that Carrboro (where I live) was not hit with the force that was predicted, but only had high winds and rain. I did get that there was a problem in Raleigh. I felt my children were OK, but my sister had something that happened, yet they were not in danger anymore so I returned to sleep.

On talking with Donna Duff in North Carolina the next morning, I found out the eye of the storm hit Carrboro the first time I was awakened and had passed over the second time I was awakened. There was not damage in Carrboro or Durham, but Raleigh had flooding and trees down. My sister had a tree fall in her yard but it did not hit her home and was a tree that they needed to take down anyway!

On reflection, I believe the hand I saw was the hand of God lifting the storm from its path and knocking the wind out! Hurricane Floyd was originally a class 5 storm and was scheduled to hit our area. Each day we prayed the storm became downgraded and its furor was altered. The shattering of glass made me realize how fragile life and property really is and can be broken. However, the pearls are symbolic of taking the rough and transforming it into another dimension of beauty which I believe we did through the meditations. From the pain and suffering others experienced we will emerge to new heights. The white cross is a way to measure and remember the impact of what was.

This is not the first time I have worked with others to spiritually connect with nature—to hear nature's message and to work with the its forces. I believe we are being told to move beyond the self to a broader awareness of our interconnectedness and the need to help each other. Storms do change course. Nature spirits will work with us to change the course of storms. We learned it in 1997 with Hurricane Fran and last year when we were threatened by yet another hurricane. I am committed to emphasize the power of prayer and focused energy with the intention to heal present disasters and share this message worldwide. As President Clinton said when he came to NC to explore the damage, "The American people are with you and have not forgotten you in your time of need." Thank you my dear friends for being there and not forgetting us.

I am reminded of the old Christmas story about the man who was so distraught that he wanted to take his life during hard times. He was given a chance to see what would have been had he not lived. He then changed and saw how much his life mattered to so many. I feel that I have been to the edge of the dimension of what could have been and didn't happen here. There is so much to be thankful for. We are blessed in love and light through shared efforts of prayers for healing.

Thank you for helping to divert the storm here at my home in North Carolina and to minimize its impact. May we continue to pray for ongoing healing of the people, land and animals who are suffering in the aftermath, especially in eastern North Carolina where the flooding is so severe.

Blessings for your help in love and light, Mary Jo.

Mary Jo Bulbrook
Carrboro, North Carolina

After the Storm

The hurricane has wrecked havoc with the lives of many here in North Carolina, especially in the eastern part of the state. The damage estimates reach into the billions. We recently had four more days of rain and the flooding has restarted. My living room wall and downstairs ceiling and wall and rug are wet—such intense rain!

Tuesday night during our local support group we did a meditation to help the flooding victims plus a Magnetic Unruffling for the east coast and Mind Clearing as well. During the time the following meditation, the following information came to Cathy Mack. I want to pass it on (see related story, "Meditation for the Animals"). I never thought of it, but this tragedy is forcing the animals and plants to raise their consciousness as was noted by Cathy. They need our help in this time of transition as well. Since Tuesday a German Shepherd has been appearing to me. I didn't know who he was or what he wanted. I told a friend last night something was up and I knew the German Shepherd had a message for me. She came to me with my two beloved pets in spirit form (Chaney and Ginger). They told me that I needed to help the animals who were in dire need. I am passing this message on to help them raise their consciousness as we are raising our consciousness as well.

The shelters are overwhelmed with misplaced pets. There is much contamination of water from dead animals. We need to raise animal spirits trapped in the aftermath of the storm and flooding. Many over-stressed animals need assistance. What I was told in my meditation during the group session is that it is important to focus on one animal group at a time and send energy out in waves of consciousness to the others. I could not focus on all animals at once. Please help us in our efforts with your focused attention to raise the animal consciousness wherever you live. They have been forgotten.

A pig also appeared to me last night and asked for help. They found many pigs stranded and sunburned badly (over 500,000 pigs were killed). Birds also came to me saying they did not have any food. These animals are part of our forgotten victims. I have cancelled my trip to South Africa next week to concentrate on the needs here: my home repairs, the focus on healing from the storm, and a new book of healing stories.

Post-Script: It's been over a month since I wrote this piece. I wanted to report that the German Shepherd that appeared to me has somehow manifested in my life. She is about one year old and her name is Maple. She was adopted in early November by my son Bill through the Independent Animal Rescue of North Carolina. Bill had put out the energy to Spirit to send her to him. Carol Komito (HT for Animals) said she is a "healer dog." I asked how you tell a healer dog and she replied, "Exactly the same way you identify healers in a classroom. They stand out as their light shines." Bill connected with his desire spiritually to find the right pet for him. The right pet for Bill called for him. I guess that's what you call healing.

Mary Jo Bulbrook
Carrboro, North Carolina

HT Community Responds to Tornado in Ohio

Early in the morning of Friday, April 9th, 1999 a tornado struck a northern suburb of Cincinnati. Four people died in the storm and 900 homes were damaged with 90-100 of those homes condemned and scheduled for demolition. A nature preserve was also destroyed. The destruction was so much worse than the pictures could ever convey. It was necessary to see it first hand to realize the power and the devastation. Pets and animals were affected as well.

What follows are the stories of some of those affected by the tornado and the work of the local Healing Touch community to respond to the needs of their community. I believe it has implications for the use of Healing Touch in disaster relief work in the future.

On Monday, April 12th, three days after the tornado struck, an Advanced Practice Healing Touch workshop was in progress here in Cincinnati. A request for volunteers to work with those affected by the tornado was circulated and 20 volunteers signed up! It was not a coincidence that we were gathered that day.

The first free clinics were held on the Friday and Saturday following the tornado. A local Methodist church a few miles south of the tornado site was more than willing to provide space for this work. About 14 people were seen those first two days (more practitioners than clients), but what stories they had to tell! We discovered that their energy fields also told the story of their experiences.

A woman whose house was unaffected while her neighbors' homes were devastated simply cried as one of the Healing Touch practitioners held her in her arms.

A young mother who brought her 5 year old twins in with her, told of the significant damage their home had sustained. One of the twins agreed to let us help him with his headache. His brother watched very intently.

Another woman came with her 10 year old son who has Down's syndrome. The young man insisted that we work on his Mom first. The mother told of how her son had saved his family. It seems he woke up before the sirens went off and alerted the rest of the family. He also took time to shut a young kitten in a bathroom. As the parents covered their children with their bodies the mother noticed he had also gathered up the family cat on the way to the basement. Their home was demolished but they and the kitten shut in the bathroom survived.

A gentleman whose roof and twin chimneys fell in on him told of finding himself in the middle of the bed and not knowing how he got there. The chimneys fell on either side of him. He suffered no broken bones or major injuries.

Several told amazing stories of angels moving them to safety. Some did not want to relive the event at all while others had a clear recollection of being picked up by the storm and spun through the air only to find themselves sitting in their front yard moments later, physically unharmed. In the early days immediately after the tornado we were really dealing with people in crisis. This is not the norm for many Healing Touch practitioners and we learned a lot about the dynamics as we worked. Energetic phrases like " blown away" and "uprooted" were commonly heard. We found Hara lines which were disrupted especially at the Tan Tien and the connection to the earth. The root chakra was frequently disturbed and we wondered how some of the people had been able to even drive to the church. We found large energy leaks in the energy fields where parts of the house had fallen on people even though they sustained little or no physical injury. Energy fields were very congested and some were displaced to one side or so drawn in that they were difficult to assess.

Practitioners used Healing Touch techniques and other advanced techniques to ground people, to reestablish and align the Hara line, to repair energy leaks, and to balance and clear the energy field. In some cases the difference was very noticeable as people walked out. One young boy was seen running and skipping in the parking lot outside the church as he left with his mother.

It became apparent that people were so occupied with meeting basic needs such as food and shelter, that it was difficult for them to take time to stop, even for 20 minutes, to breathe and relax. It was evident that the healing process for those affected by the storm would continue for some time into the future. In cooperation with a local Catholic church very near the devastated area, local Healing Touch practitioners continued to offer Healing Touch twice a month through August 1999. More than 35 clients received more than 100 Healing Touch sessions at these clinics from more than 23 Healing Touch volunteers over the next four months.

The evening sessions at the church actually became a kind of support network for the "Tornado Victors" as they became known. They developed a pattern of gathering at the start of the session and spent time with each other as they waited their turn for Healing Touch. We continued to see energetic effects similar to those we had seen immediately after the tornado, especially with first time clients.

Many of the clients related concerns about their pets. Carol Komitor just happened to be scheduled to be in Cincinnati for a Healing Touch for Animals class in June. Coincidence? I don't think so! Carol stayed over an extra day and held a free clinic with other practitioners for pets affected by the tornado. Our interconnectedness never was more apparent for many of us involved. The earth, the animals, the trees, and the humans were all in need of healing.

We learned much from this experience. For example, we learned about the difficulty of documenting our work in a consistent manner, the need to attend to small children as we worked on their parents, dealing with people in crisis, how to organize this kind of effort on an urgent and ongoing basis, and when to begin teaching self-care.

On the evening of the second to the last session of the clinics, we met with the group and explained that it was time for them to continue the healing process on their own. That evening we taught several self-care techniques for them to use. They were eager to learn. A list of Healing Touch practitioners was also distributed.

On the last evening, the Parish Nurse and the Tornado Victors gave each of the Healing Touch volunteers a certificate of appreciation and a Blessing Bag with several aromatherapy candles. The Blessing Bag works like this. You are instructed to write down your blessings and put them in your Blessing Bag. The instructions promise that, "soon it will be full to overflowing."

The opportunity to work with the Tornado Victors was truly a blessing for all of us. There is a place and a need for energy work and Healing Touch in the aftermath of natural disasters. We need to be prepared to respond in the future.

I want to acknowledge and thank all the Greater Cincinnati Healing Touch practitioners who responded so generously when called. I also want to acknowledge Mary Jo Bulbrook, Janet Mentgen, and all those in the Healing Touch community for their support and encouragement as we summoned the courage and the energy to offer our services.

Mary M. Duennes
Cincinnati, Ohio

Littleton Crisis in Colorado: The Whole World is Watching

On April 20th, 1999 two high school students opened fire during lunch at Columbine High School in Littleton, Colorado killing one teacher and 17 students in addition to themselves. Soon the panic and fear spread over the whole school, community, city, and state. Parents and students stayed home for days glued to or avoiding the TV reports. The news, and consequently the fear and panic, spread across the nation. By the weekend it had spread across the globe. I first received phone calls from shocked family members, then friends across the U.S. and finally e-mails with calls from friends as far away as Australia and New Zealand.

This demonstrates how small our world has gotten. News travels fast, and traumatic news the fastest. The physics principal is that all things are interactive as all is energy. What I am about to report is related to that principle.

In Denver, spring had arrived before that April day. By the very next day we had bitter cold weather again and within two days we had snow. For the next two weeks we alternated between rain, snow and sleet. It remained cold and the sun did not shine (except for brief moments) for two solid weeks. With the cold, gloomy weather came depression.

Two healing sessions were done by Healing Touch practitioners on the land "outside" the Columbine High School library using a technique called, "Healing Earth Trauma" (see the next story). This was a global effort with healers linking first locally, then nationally and finally (via e-mail) globally. Ten Healing Touch sessions were also done for Jefferson County School administrators on the trauma team responsible for dealing with the press, the police, and calling families to verify whereabouts of the students and teachers that day. The healing sessions were a volunteer effort by Healing Touch practitioners within the local Denver community.

By the end of the second week as the heavy energy was starting to clear, the sun returned to our skies and the temperatures again reached late spring levels. I believe the difference I felt was made by the effort put forth with love by the global healing community. We worked to release fear and panic, build cleansing energies and anchor it locally, spread compassion and forgiveness, and hold the space for healing across the globe. The laws of physics which speaks to the interconnectedness of all things shows us that we indeed make a difference in others lives. Trauma is not only held in the human heart, it is held and spread by the earth and her other inhabitants through the invisible bond of energy. The work we did here was to clear energetic trauma from the physical space locally, and then send it out radiantly, to include the community and eventually the world. It created a path to assist in healing for all those whose lives were touched by this traumatic event.

What we did, can and needs to be repeated whenever there is trauma in an area. Remember trauma is stored energetically not only in individuals, but in the environment as well. Reach out and touch your community with peace and love.

Janna Moll
Highlands Ranch, Colorado

Earth Trauma Healing

In order to assist with healing the earth that had been traumatized by the tragic events that took place at Columbine High School, a group of three Healing Touch Practitioners accompanied me on April 25, 1999 to perform a powerful earth healing. The technique of Healing Earth Trauma originated with Sally Clements, a certified HT Practitioner in Dayton, Ohio. This was given to her to aid in the healing of individuals. It was modified through guidance to promote healing of the earth as all things are interconnected. In addition to the four practitioners located in Littleton, CO, Sally in Ohio and Jean Gustafson in upstate New York simultaneously performed the process, linking together the three sources as well as with other healers from around the globe via the Internet. The task of the group was to hold the energy for this healing work. Energetically it was extremely powerful for all involved!

As we approached Columbine High School from Clement Park, a memorial service was just finishing. Five thousand people had attended including the mayor, senators, the vice president of the U.S. and others. Even so, we were undisturbed.

It was a very cold and rainy day about 6:00 p.m. Denver time. Before starting, the three with me in Littleton drew energetic pictures of the area. I performed the technique while standing inside a triangle formed by Terry Terry, Carole Brush and Dave Rourke. The process took 40 minutes. All involved from across the world reported amazing and interesting experiences as we later connected together by e-mail.

Some reported the sky full of small white candles, the Archangels were present and "time and space" seemed to be altered. Some (linked by the Internet) saw the location very vividly in their awareness, even the inside of the school. All saw a vortex of energy form and disband over the school where we were. The energy shift was felt very profoundly by all of us on that cold evening.

The technique was repeated on a later date with Carol Komitor in Longmont, Colorado linked with me at Columbine High School and both performing the technique simultaneously. This event was unbelievably sad for me. Much pain and suffering was released from this spot on the Earth. Near the end of the technique I was aware of a line of young people filing past me into the light. One young woman stood next to me looking extremely lost and scared. I encouraged her repeatedly to move into the light with her friends. Finally she did, turning around and looking at me again with very sad and lost looking eyes. I surrounded her with love as she and the others moved down a light-drenched corridor. A peace came over the athletic field and area of Columbine High School when I finished. It was the first warm, sunny day since that fateful day.

Afterward I saw a picture of the young woman who had been standing next to me that day. She was one of two girls killed at Columbine. I was surprised. I guess I never really thought I would bridge this event with facts, yet there she was again! She looked so self-assured and happy in the photo on TV and I remembered feeling very close to her family following the shootings. They embodied the same beliefs as I about forgiveness and peace. Very powerful words in light of their grief, loss, and pain!

Energy work is on the one hand very vague. It occupies a gray area that science hasn't yet fully understood and embraced. However, we who have experienced it know its power and potential. I know that I made a difference in at least one person's life over the course of those two healings. I ask you to trust that you too have the ability to forever touch the lives of others.

Janna Moll
Highlands Ranch, Colorado

Journey into the Light: Walking the Labyrinth

In 1996 in Denver, HT was sponsoring a joint venture of walking a canvas replication of the Chartres Cathedral Labyrinth. A Labyrinth is an archetype, a divine imprint related to religious traditions in various forms throughout the world. It is a way of going inside to gain insight and move from the distractions of the world to our inner life. The center is a place of prayer and meditation to receive clarity about our lives. As we walk back out on the same path that brought us in, we are granted the power to act. The walk is a shared journey, an activity that communities can do together to coalesce and unify vision.

My experience was another one of the "feelings" that got activated and stirred within me. I knew I would be doing something with a Labyrinth. The canvas replication was designed to be carried to workshop to workshop to introduce this ancient form of meditation in places where there was no Labyrinth. The original idea is to have a land Labyrinth usually in a garden providing integration with nature.

My immediate response was that a Labyrinth was a tool that could provide self-directed psychotherapy for a person. I then wondered how to integrate this tool with what I know about psychotherapy, energy work, and gardens. I came home motivated and contacted a friend who has a spiritual connection with plants and animals.

He quickly resonated to my idea and we soon brought into focus doing a garden replication of the Chartres Cathedral labyrinth like the one that I had walked in Denver. Six months went by and nothing came together. On New Year's Eve Donna Duff and I were invited to Cathy Mack's house for the holiday with a plan to walk a garden Labyrinth in Raleigh, NC that was a rough replication of the Chartres Cathedral Labyrinth.

We arrived late at the garden and had to climb a fence in a drizzling rain to walk the labyrinth. As we did excitement mounted. A vision of a Labyrinth came to me that was based on the seven chakras and the energy field. I first saw an X. In the Runes, X stands for partnerships and since that is the name of my business I felt that was very important. Then a I saw a box drawn around the X that divided the area into a square. This represented to me the divisions of body, mind, emotion, and spirit. Then I saw an image of seven concentric circles that represented the aura. The point where each of the circles met the X formed the chakras. This was depicted as a small circle with an X in at the intersection. A circle with and X in it is an ancient symbol used for protection of the chakras. Making the vision three-dimensional formed a pyramid. By collapsing the X into a line it formed a Hara connecting the person to the Divine and the center of the earth. This then became a time dimensional line of energy that a person could travel back in time through all ages!

I was so excited after the walk and couldn't wait to tell Cathy and Donna what came to me. When we went back to Cathy's home I drew the vision and it was named, "Journey into the Light, to promote Energetic Healing through walking the Pyramid Labyrinth."

There is no set way to walk it, like there is with the Chartres Cathedral Labyrinth. You just do it. In the doing it, you then open the consciousness wherever you are. The size of the Labyrinth does not matter, only that it is a perfect square.

Some walk straight into the center. Others walk around the edges. Some stay in a particular dimension, the chakras, the field or body, emotion, mind or spirit. Remember, there is no set way to do it. Following your awareness, or lack thereof, is what is intended. Changes occur both in and out of awareness. This is not something that is forced, it just happens or it doesn't!

The Labyrinth is also laid out with spirit in the north, emotion in the east, physical in the south, and mental in the west. I have found that when others walk it with you like what is done in a workshop, one becomes aware of the energy of the other person and how one resonates or doesn't resonate to another's energy. This is also a clue regarding one's own energy. It is a spiritual tool of transformation. It is as spiritual as it gets based on what is right for a person at a point in time.

The intention was to make a garden one that could be easily replicated in an area based on the natural topography, and local plant life. Hence when a person walked it, they would go back into time, related to the land and be changed as they worked through the energy of the unfinished business from that time frame. A person not as advanced, however, would only experience it at the depth of the awareness that they could achieve.

With this in mind, I set out to create a canvas Labyrinth based on the design that was channeled to me and establish workshops throughout the world to teach the replication of this process that could be a self-healing tool for personal transformation. The man in Carrboro, NC who I commissioned to make the canvas labyrinth looked at me in disbelief when I described the purpose of the project and why I was making it. When I picked up the canvas about two weeks later, (it was a 12 foot square version), the first thing he said to me is that he was not sure he would give it back to me. I stopped in my tracks and asked why. He told me he painted this in his home in the living room, as he did not have any other place to do it. He removed all the furniture in the room, laid out the canvas, and proceeded to paint what was my vision. He sat on it, laid on it, crawled on it for two weeks and was never happier in his life. I looked at his wife who also worked with him and she silently nodded her head yes! I knew then if the Journey into the Light Labyrinth could transform a skeptic who had no intention of it doing anything, then there was power in it! This was proven time and time again as others began to walk this new design, based on the nature of the energy system of the human being as outlined by spirit.

It was introduced on the tour in 1997 and since that time others have been taught how to lead the workshops. A laminated one was made so that a person could use it for problem solving by walking the Labyrinth with their fingers. The workshops I have held so far have confirmed my vision that indeed it is a powerful tool to take people back in time and have them complete healing that then affects the here and now. Some had clear visions of the past lifetimes. Those who that concept was foreign to did not experience it in the same way. One goes only as far as the individual perspective allows one to go.

A picture of the Labyrinth appears in the photograph section. As with other things that have come to me, the power of something is only realized as people have experiences and report them. In the beginning I did not record the findings, as this is only one of the many things that I am involved in. In Houston, San Francisco, Detroit, and Carrboro we have ongoing experiences with the Labyrinth. It also has been used in New Zealand. More stories will be given in other volumes as time goes on. So welcome to a Journey into the Light back into time! In closing I would like to share a few comments from some of the participants who have walked it:

Clearing (Sister Barbara Cavanaugh)
My experience in Walking the Labyrinth is that it is another effective tool in self-healing. I see that I may focus in on where I am in my life as a whole at the moment, using the chakras and auras in my intent to clear, balance and fill with energetic healing and reach my highest potential as a person and healer. This process also gives opportunity and space which can bring closure to long-standing personal issues that lead to a totally new perspective. It sharpened my awareness of who I am and what is expected of me, and in short, insight into how to live life.

Listening (Jeff Kemp)
I found myself focused immediately and benefiting from the Labyrinth as a tool. It seemed that once my intent was set, I was guided. My first steps acted to clear out my left brain surges. Then a purity of thought or input from outside myself emerged. I asked a question with each step and received clear prompt answers that cut right through to the heart to my issues. This was a very nurturing experience.

Following (Mary L. Klinger)
This past weekend a friend and I were camping along a stream in the foothills of Mount Whitney in the Eastern Sierras. We were exchanging healing techniques and practicing. With treat excitement I gave her a copy of the laminated Journey into the Light Labyrinth. We sat with our feet in the stream working through it with our fingers. We then moved to the land where I proceeded to share some Healing Touch with her. I finished a sequence on her and then it was my turn for a "treatment." At the end I told her to how reassess the field with a hand scan. She remarked that her hands were being pulled or drawn towards my feet. We both looked down to "see," with our intuitive sight, my energy trailing off my feet straight towards the water. Our first thought was that for some reason it was wanting something from the water. Then it became clear. It went to where I was with the Labyrinth. Something was not quite done and it needed to reconnect to finish the process. It did complete with this awareness for another three minutes by using the labyrinth. This is truly powerful tool of connection, process, and enlightenment.

Integrating (Kia Abilay)
The meditation set the tone and I received some direction in my mind's eye. When I started walking it brought a whole set of emotional experiences from my lifetime and connected it to my present physical and emotional self. It also gave me a healing process and reassurance from my guides on some self-healing techniques that I am not alone in this journey! It was an incredible healing experience. Thank you!

The Power of Love (Eileen Herbst)
I began the Labyrinth experience by asking the question: "Where do I start?" In reply I heard, "Your Heart." I entered the Labyrinth and went to the West/North corner, which is also the mental/emotional corner and focused on openness. I found myself walking up the chakras and hearing a message at each one:

1) Root or sensing: "All cultures are connected and are one, they are also tied to nature."

2) Sacral or feeling: "Everyone is my family."

3) Mental or thinking: "Use your power for others."

4) Heart or loving: "Just be."

5) Throat / hearing: "Speak lovingly to all even your 'enemies,' who are really your teachers."

6) Brow / seeing: "Set your mind on love."

7) Crown / knowing: "Love guides the world."

I stepped off into the North corner of the mental quadrant and heard the words of Julian of Norwich: "All shall be well and all manner of things shall be well." I stood there a little longer and another message was heard: "Speak your truth honestly." Then pain was experienced in my breast/heart area. I walked to the physical corner and did a Pain Drain and Unruffling. I walked back to the center of the Labyrinth and the message, "Seek Peace," concluded my experience.

Conclusion (Mary Jo Bulbrook)

The messages that Eileen got for the chakras will now become part of Journey to the Light. Her experience represents the Way to the Light in human processes. This experience which occurred in November, 1999 in Detroit, Michigan will set the tone for a renewed sense of connection to God in our journey. Another focus was added at this time inspired by Joan Borysenko's *Pocketful of Miracles*, 1994. The archangels were invoked to support the work. Journey to the Light is now guided by:

St. Uriel, the Light (or fire) of God related to clarity, rebirth and new beginnings (East and Spring);

St. Gabriel, the Strength of God related to energy to support and overcome fear, bringing the divine into manifestation (South and Summer);

St. Raphael, Healer of God, related to death and rebirth, transcending opposites into wholeness (West and Fall);

St. Michael, like unto God related to the energy of wisdom and love (North and Winter).

7 | CONNECTING WITH GUIDANCE

Development of the Healer

Becoming a Healer

Be open

And know

That the Source

Is ever ready

To be there for you

As you merge your spirits together.

Mary Jo Bulbrook
Carrboro, North Carolina
(January 8, 1997)

My Personal Journey: Mary Jo Bulbrook

"What are you doing up in the middle of the night? It is 3:00 a.m. and you should be asleep!"

"I am sorry to disturb you mom, but I can't sleep," I said. I was pacing the floor in our kitchen in my family's home in Cincinnati, Ohio. I was very focused but confused. "I think I am suppose to be a nurse and go to Mount St. Joseph," I said. "I keep getting a feeling I need to do this and don't know why."

"Go back to bed, that's foolishness," mom said. She left me wandering in the house and was perplexed by my sudden change to go into nursing without a rationale. I could not understand what was happening to me, but somehow I never doubted the awareness. I knew I would make plans to do exactly what I was sensing.

It was the summer of 1962, one and a half months before I was to start college. I was enrolled at Villa Madonna College in Kentucky as a physics major. Mom had wanted me to go to Mount St. Joseph, which was ten miles from our home in Cincinnati, Ohio. I had not wanted to go there. About six months previously I had said to my friends when we were discussing what we were planning to do after high school, "The last thing in the world I want to do is become a nurse!" Now I was making a 360-degree turn in my life's career and changing my destiny over a "feeling awareness" without rationale. This decision was to set the course for the future of my life and the beginning of following guidance.

I attended Mount St. Joseph having been accepted into the nursing program by a reluctant Director of the School of Nursing who informed me that they usually do not accept last minute enrollments. She seemed to make her decision after she questioned me about my high school activities. I said that I was a member of the National Honor Society. After I said that she did not hesitate, which was so unusual since before that she was very hesitant. Sister immediately made plans for me to attend the Mount and arranged for me to receive a National Institute of Mental Health Training Scholarship. The interesting part of this is that I was only in the Honor Society for one semester, and very surprised when I made it after all these years. I am not exactly an academic "giant," but rather ordinary. I had a mild case of dyslexia which was undetected at that time. I took the acceptance at Mt. St. Joseph to be yet another sign in of the role of Spirit in my destiny.

In my second year of college, I have another "night awakening" and am "told" by that same vague feeling or awareness, I am to do spiritual work. To me that meant being a nun and I knew, they got that wrong! I forgot about the experience until 30 years later when I looked back over my life and saw the pattern that emerged. I realized that indeed I am doing spiritual work although not as a nun!

From about 1964 to 1972 my life followed the normal course. I finished college, worked as a nurse at Cincinnati's Children's Hospital, and got married. I then completed a masters degree, moved to Texas, started a family, and began my teaching career at Tarrant County Junior College in Ft. Worth, Texas. Within a year I started a doctoral program in nursing. My life was very active and full. I occasionally would experience synchronicity in events that made me stop to think and see the power of the unknown, but the voices did not become clear until I moved with my family to Utah. I was picked by Madeline Leininger, renowned nursing professor, to head up the Psychiatric Mental Health Program at the University of Utah being responsible for the masters and doctoral psychiatric nursing program. I settled into my career as a "traditional academic."

Then in 1972 one of my psychiatric nursing colleagues introduced me to the world of the newly emerging paradigm of "holistic health." That introduction was the beginning of the next phase of my life and started me on the road to fulfill the destiny of doing "spiritual work" originally charted in 1964.

I had started becoming involved with the teachings and work of Virginia Satir, internationally renowned family therapist. She and I became close associates. She mentored me and took me under her wing. The work of Spirit became very prominent in my relationship and connection with Virginia. The voices returned directing and predicting what was to come. The synchronicity in my life became too apparent to not notice something was happening. However I was still naive at this point, doubting the real significance of my life plans unfolding.

Virginia was very spiritual in her approach in caring for people. She set a new course in the field of mental health, one shaped by early childhood experiences and family dynamics. Virginia's work then and now is considered "magic" as she could accomplish things many others couldn't. She would get the clients no one else had success with and change their lives. Over the years I was to discover

Virginia's "magic" was a deep spiritual connection and trust in the intrinsic good of all human beings. This philosophy and mentoring directly shaped the work that I do today and the way it is done. The "magic" of energy work is not unlike what Virginia was doing without calling it holistic. Virginia was one of the original holistic practitioners and leaders in this movement. I believe the success of her therapy was the energy changes she initiated with the client through her way of being, her way of touching verbally and non-verbally, through a loving, gentle, non-invasive, spiritual energy connection.

The details of my work with Virginia is yet another story to be told. Later in this book, there is some material (Transforming and Healing the Self) that tells part of my "Satir story" and how it shapes the healing work I am doing today. For now, I will refocus on other factors in my development as a healer.

In 1980 I "know" my work is completed in Utah. However, I did not have any sense of what was next. I had quit my job at the university without having secured another position. I was becoming agitated, as various jobs I would interview for would suddenly disappear without rhyme or reason. In February, four months before my job would end, I was a single mother with three sons to support. Suddenly the voices return and I am told that where I am to go next is not ready yet. I was told not to worry, as I would be taken care of. Oddly enough, as I shared this awareness with my friends, I experienced a sense of calm and patience and believed that I *would* be taken care of!

One day in May I was sitting in the office of a colleague at the University of Utah when he received a phone call from the Director of Nursing at Memorial University of Newfoundland in Canada who was looking for faculty in psychiatric mental health nursing. She asked my friend if he knew anyone looking for a position. He laughed, looked at me and said, "Yes and she is sitting here in my office right now." He handed the phone to me. The director interviewed me briefly, invited me to come to Memorial University in June for an interview. By August I had moved to Newfoundland which is in the far northeastern point of Canada. I became Professor in Nursing and Coordinator of the Graduate Program in Nursing at Memorial University of Newfoundland within a very short time.

I had left the United States kicking and screaming. "I do not want to leave the country of my birth. Where am I being let to and why? It's not fair! I don't want to leave my children with their dad in Texas for a year till I get settled." I had no other choice or so it seemed. I felt strong guidance about this decision to move to Newfoundland. But, once again I couldn't fully understand the reason so I was in mental turmoil over the uncertainty of it all. Although I felt spiritually aligned it did not help my mental or emotional state. From this experience I learned a key principle in spiritual direction: *You may know something is right spiritually but emotionally or mentally you are the pits.*

It wasn't until years later, looking back, I can see how those experiences once again shaped my spiritual calling and guidance. I am reporting this detail so that others will be comforted when they reach the a similar point in their lives—*doubt and chaos when faced with the choice to follow guidance or not.*

In Utah I had pursued a traditional career of academic excellence and leadership. On the side I pursued my interests in holistic medicine and alternative therapies, never understanding how I would incorporate this training into my established career. However this lack of insight did not deter me. I only followed what I was led to and had a sense of was right for me, many times with the discouragement of family and peers. This taught me another principle of spiritual direction: *Others may not support your decisions.*

I had studied Therapeutic Touch with Dolores Krieger in 1976 in San Francisco. This experience set in motion another influence that significantly shaped my present work. Also I studied energy medicine with John Thie, the creator of Touch For Health and a colleague in the Virginia Satir Network. Touch For Health is energy meridian work born out of the John's chiropractic profession that also incorporated applied kinesiology with energy work. With this modality I began formally introducing to my professional contacts and lay public the power of doing energy work with clients. However, this holistic work still was on the fringe of my career, as I still did not have a clue or inclination to leave what I was doing as an academic. I loved my work and was very good at it. Still I continued to pursue my interest, *subtly being led spiritually*—another principle in the development of the healer.

I first began using the title "healer" at Memorial University. The School of Nursing under my leadership offered a workshop titled, "Health and Healing in the Future," that included Virginia Satir, Gordon Stokes the international training director of Touch For Health, and myself. The publicity for that workshop marked the first time I formally used the title of "healer." The Director of Nursing, my supervisor, summoned me into her office to inform me that the Vice-President of Academic Affairs told her I was not to use the title "healer."

I claimed my power and stated, "That is what I do and what I am. I will not disclaim the title 'healer.'" That was the first and last time I was challenged in my university career using the designated title of "healer." *All healers will some day need to own up to the title and withstand the influence of being challenged in the use of that title, whether it is from family, friends or colleagues.*

Having established a firm commitment to being a healer I began to realize that I no longer desired to do what I was doing. It was now time to be something different than being a university Professor. I was becoming more and more committed to energy-based healing and teaching people how to do that for themselves and for others.

The next major event to shape my destiny as a healer was the realization that although I knew a lot about mental and physical health from the holistic perspective, I now wanted to learn more about spiritual care and other dimensions of reality. It was a conscious decision to move beyond where I was, into the unknown

Ever since 1970 I had a private nursing practice to compliment my nursing university career. I believed then and now, if one is to be a successful teacher, she/he needs to be an expert in what was taught from a grass roots level. Hence the stimulus to develop and maintain an active practice. It was through that practice that I began to incorporate all the holistic things I was learning. In that role I could go beyond the definition of who and what I was and to where I wanted to go.

I continually maintained my spiritual focus asking to be guided to my life's path. It was prayer and meditation that set my course, not experiences of formalized religion that I felt failed me and others as their humanness at times blocked their connection to the Light.

As I offered alternative therapies, I was becoming known as an expert in the local healing community. I increased my prayers and the voices returned. The final step in my clearly linking to Spirit was formed.

I remember very clearly the changes that began when I started a support group for cancer patients, their family, friends, and health care professionals. One of my students, who I had helped when she lost her husband to cancer and was a Master's degree student at Memorial, said she was now ready to explore holistic health. Up to that time being a "scientific person in mind," she was doubtful of the benefits of the intuitive nature of the holistic movement.

After the first session of a group therapy she attended, I was riding with my children and Donna Duff to the local movie theatre. While driving a man appeared to me and left the impression he was my student's deceased husband. I told Donna I thought he wanted to get a message to his wife through me.

I felt that I was loosing my mind. I was very unsure of what I just said. Nonetheless, on Sunday I called up my student and told her about my experience. Being a skeptic, she listened patiently but without acceptance until I gave her the following information. I described the man who appeared to me stating he had brown hair and I thought he was her husband. "Oh no, he did not have brown hair. It turned grey very early," she said.

"Did he have brown hair though when young?" I asked. She paused and said, "Yes." Then when I focused on connecting with the energy that appeared while driving a few days earlier, I was given the information he had a very prominent chest that one would remark about. My student admitted that was true but still was doubtful. I connected again and was told that he was 5'8". She confirmed this was true.

Both of us were in awe of the conversation and hung up in bewilderment about what this may mean. At the next group session the following week, her husband again "appeared" to me in the group. I called attention to what I was seeing as it happened in class. He showed me a scene of his wedding with her. It was in a meadow, outside and not in a church. She had flowers in her hair and was very happy. The student was astounded that I described in detail her wedding that I could not have had knowledge of. I then heard Gene Kelly singing and dancing to "Singing in the Rain." I laughed and told her that there must be some mistake as that music was from my generation and not the student who was about ten years my junior. She said very seriously, "That is my favorite song."

Without a doubt she and I knew that I had tapped into the spirit of her husband who had died several years earlier. I had never met him but only supported my student during his dying process. They had gone all over the world for treatment to cure his cancer, but were unsuccessful. Once it was established without a doubt that he was her husband in both her and my mind, he said very gently, "Tell her that I am OK and was not meant to live long on the earth. Who she was with now is meant to be her life partner, not him. He was very pleased that she was with him and wanted her to know that." We were both stunned. With that information, the cycle was complete. He never appeared to me again. That was the start of my not only hearing "voices," but knowing that discarnate spirits came to me to help others with their healing.

I had never before experienced connecting directly with Spirit, although I have often felt inspired and led. Not knowing what to do with this experience, I just "lived" with it—not in fear, not in awe, but just lived with it.

Over the next few years, I would soon learn how to connect with Spirit and use that connection for my client's healing. I did not want my evolved gifts as a healer to be, "Look into the crystal ball and tell me if I am going to meet Mr. Right." No, that is not what I was about. I wanted to focus my intuitive abilities with God to help others in their healing. Another principle in the development of the healer: *We can determine how ones' gifts will be used. The healer is not a passive recipient of the influence of an outside spirit, but "co-creates" together with the client a reality that will help in the healing of a person.*

At this point I reached a point of no return. I will never doubt that other realities do exist and they can be accessed given the calling, and answering of the call by a committed healer.

No, I am not crazy. Yes, I have moved into alternative realities, beyond anything I had learned in my nursing career or career as an academic with a recognized doctorate degree in teaching. *My truth was now real, and I would never return to the ordinary again.*

The path of my role as a healer and teacher of healers was well established in 1986. I was becoming less and less interested in academic life and committed to move into the holistic movement full time. The question became: Where are the jobs? How do I support three children and myself? What will others say about my intuitive abilities? Have I gone too far with no return, or had I reached the peak of the next phase of my development as a healer?

Mary Jo Bulbrook
Carrboro, North Carolina

Evolution as a Healer: Barbara Harris

Very early in my life I discovered that my hands were able to soothe members of my family and friends that were hurting. At 17 years of age Spirit provided me with an unsolicited full scholarship to study nursing. This was a blessing as there was only enough family funds to send my twin brother to college. Many people confirmed what I suspected. I was told repeatedly that my touch was the "best medicine." Now, of course, I know that this is not unique. I used touch frequently as a student nurse in the early fifties because at times I did not know what else to do to comfort a hurting or dying patient.

In the early seventies I was introduced to the body of work developed at New York University by Dolores Krieger known as Therapeutic Touch (TT). After using TT on a quadriplegic patient and having him report that he "felt something" and observing his leg spasms lessen, my intellectual curiosity was aroused! I studied TT with both Dr. Krieger and her early students. I practiced and taught Therapeutic Touch for over ten years. This knowledge served to whet my appetite to learn other energy/touching methods and led to my initiation as a Reiki Master/Teacher and a licensed massage therapist. I also continued to study many healing cultures such as the Native American and Shamanism, and advanced body work methods such as Cranio-Sacral, reflexology, and acupressure.

While serving as President of the National Association of Nurse Massage Therapists, I learned of the diversity and outstanding content of the Healing Touch Program. I introduced it as a facilitator to my area of the west coast of Florida. To date, I have completed Level I, IIA, and IIB. Though I wish to continue my studies for HT Certification my pathway has taken a turn when I was called by the Blessed Mother to write a book (*Conversations With Mary*) that was published in May of 1999. Deciding to devote full time to the book, Spirit had other plans. After a wonderful traveling summer, I was challenged with a frontal brain tumor that was removed in August of 1999. Thankfully this tumor was benign, so I continue my journey of experiencing first-hand what it means to be a patient and also to surrender to a Higher Power.

Barbara Harris
Osprey, Florida

CONNECTING WITH VIRGINIA SATIR

Transforming and Healing the Self

As we nearly finished compiling the *Healing Stories* book, I was compelled to search through some old files for reasons beyond my understanding. In this process I came across a booklet I put together in 1989 after the death of Virginia Satir, the world-renowned healer and pioneer in family therapy, who was one of my mentors, teachers, and dear friends. The booklet is titled, *Transforming and Healing the Self*, and was written to assist me and my friends with our grieving process on losing Virginia. It was also the start of my awareness of receiving clear guidance from Virginia from the other side to help me in my healing work.

Virginia and I had a very special relationship that was closely linked to both to our mutual interests in holistic health. Most of the new things I learned to do that were energy-based, I first did them on Virginia. We would spend many hours talking about energy work. She shared her fears about "What will people think if I let them know what I am interested in?" You have to understand, this was the middle 70's and the beginning days of "legitimate" professionals studying the implications of energy work in the healing realm. I would often challenge her and say what was important to do is what she was being guided to do and not what other people thought! Imagine me therapizing the therapist!

What I was to later discover after 10 years, I am now carrying on her work with a focus of energy-based healing. She predicted that I would be doing this, often telling me that I would follow in her footsteps. The material that follows marks that transition. I am including a portion of it in the Healing Stories Book for several reasons: 1) it is a story tied into some of the most important experiences in my life, especially in my development as a healer, and 2) it shares knowledge about helping individuals and families change and heal that I think is important to reflect on.

Virginia is one of the key influences of my philosophy about health and healing. This book would not be complete without her teachings in it, as the process of healing is channeled through me from her mentorship. As I reread the Dedication to that 1989 publication, it is now a decade later. That book was written during the same time of the year that all my important experiences happened with Virginia. So it is no surprise I revisited that time frame this year completely out of conscious awareness. As reread this booklet while in the middle of creating a new book on healing stories, I believe Virginia was guiding me to get her material in the new book! I had forgotten about this material and now realize, especially since it is a spiritual guide, her material wants to come forward.

Enjoy the following excerpts from, *Transforming and Healing the Self: A Guide to Spiritual Awakening* that was inspired and influenced by Virginia Satir. This guide to spiritual awakening was developed 10 years ago to help one achieve a level of heightened consciousness; to build or rebuild the you, who you want to be, shedding the old self that no longer is needed or wanted. The old self is the self that was created and raised by the parents and other influential persons in your life. The new self is the adult you, reparenting those aspects of the child within that need to be healed in order to become who you were more fully meant to be.

In this day of adult children from dysfunctional families or other addictive behaviors there is an urgent need to transform and heal the self. What seems to be happening in these situations is that there is a void in knowledge and nurturing experiences. This occurs because the parents, while doing the best they could, were not fully able to produce vibrantly alive children who were acknowledged for just Being rather than for Doing to please others.

The answer to this need for growth and change is individual and lies deep within the self. To reach this depth requires the ability to access inner and outer levels of consciousness available to all human beings. Hence the following material is designed to trigger that internal self-reflective process.

Transforming and Healing the Self is influenced by my seven-teen-year journey with Virginia Satir. As the coordinator of the first "process community" in Park City, Utah in 1982 of the Avanta Network, Virginia's International Teaching Group, I have seen the ongoing dynamic influence for growth and change take place throughout the world. My goal is to spread what I know about strengthening spiritual development in individuals as the cornerstone of all change and growth. Physical and mental healing occurs as the spiritual dimensions is awakened and developed. Western medicine including physical and mental health/illness care has little knowledge and experience in spiritual development and care.

In journeying throughout life, the process from Being to Becoming is the purpose of life, uniting the Lower Self to the Higher Self through the Heart Center. We were not meant to be controlled or manipulated by others. Rather those in our charge are given seeds for growth. Growth and change is guided through you in the day by day, year by year progression from one level to another. The responsibility to change and grow, ultimately rests with the individual charged with the destiny of the self. Other influences such as parents, friends, teachers, bosses are only guideposts or roadblocks that need to be tasted, explored, and digested, thus keeping only that which supports healthy vibrant life!

Mary Jo Bulbrook
Carrboro, NC

INNER REFLECTIONS

Conflict
Know that I am with you.
Your have been a big help to me
Although I have not always acknowledged or known it.
The conflict between us was necessary in order for you to separate.
Allow yourself to continue to grow and be
All you were destined to be.

Joy
Life is meant to be joyful.
I joy
In your joy!

Eliminate Slavery
You must free yourself from the demands of others.
That is your first lesson on earth.
We were meant to be
Helpers, Supporters, Builders,
Not slaves! Some of your distress and illness is
From excessive clinging of others' expectations on you.
Free the self from oppression of all kinds!

Uniting Soft and Strong
Be as the oak.
Stand firm and strong
While adding the bending of the willow tree.

The combination of uniting the two forces
Of strong and soft
Will produce a force unmatched on earth.
We were meant to be
Both male and female in abilities.

For to have new life
Each is essential
To create a Human Being
Not a Human Becoming!

Trust Your Inner Self
Journey well my friend
And learn to trust
Your inner self more!

Lesson
In the earth plane there are lessons given to direct the path of
The emerging and budding new soul.
Free will directs that path.
Other people can be a healing beam of life-giving energy or life-
taking energy.
Learn to determine the differences in you life's experiences!

Come to Me
Bring me into you heart
And I will serve you
Once again.

Process to Find Your Truth
Be aware of self-serving interests that try to manifest themselves
And those whose ideas are not from the heart.
How can you tell if these criteria are met or not?
First, take in the information and meditate on it.
Then take the input into your heart.
If it feels right, even if it seems grandiose or simple,
Then it is right for that moment in time.
Progress to the next step and when you feel shaky as you progress,
again take the data inside.
Meditate on it, run it through you whole being and the truth and
Rightness will ring true.
There is a process of trust at stake here.
Mountains can be moved when truth is on your side.
Truth is not self-serving but rather that which serves the Spirit/God
And the Higher Self!

Radiate Inner Glow and Outer Light
Radiate In and Out
Your Inner Glow and Outer Light.
And you will find
Your life will become
More how you want it to be
And were destined to be!

Guides
There are three guides I leave with you.
Peace Within,
Peace Between,
Peace Among.
Inherent in achieving the above you will achieve great things.
For it is in clearing out the self of harmful present and past energy.
That who we were more beautifully intended to be, has the opportunity to be manifested. This process and new state of being can solve problems, issues that occur between and among people of all nations and persuasions!

Based on connections with Virginia Satir
Mary Jo Bulbrook (1989)

GUIDED READINGS TO GROW AND CHANGE

This section includes readings and healing inspirations that came from the various Energetic Healing courses I have taught. As you read them, the ones that resonate to you are related to your need to grow and change. Meditate on the ones that attune to your energy. You will know deep inside what is needed for your personal healing.

I started doing what I call "readings" years ago as messages started coming to me in my work as a healer. I realized how important these messages were to individuals in their healing, so I decided to adopt a philosophy to do a reading for everyone in the class if I could because I knew everyone wanted something for himself or herself in healing!

When others started teaching EH, they said, that there is no way they could do readings. Then without expecting it, Bernie Clarke, the International Training Director of EH announced to me that she was going to try to learn how to do readings. Within a short time, she was doing readings very successful from feedback from the students! I said, if one can do it, then the possibility exists for others to do it. Soon I was requiring the other EH teacher to try doing readings. After most of then got over their fear of being inadequate, soon the messages started coming, slowly at first, then with speed and clarity. Everyone was able to get readings! It goes to show when you expand your framework of possibilities, new things can happen.

I have used this same process regarding teaching first my faculty how to do aura drawings and increase their visual clues to tap into Higher Sense Perception. Everyone has expanded his or her capacity by trying! *It only takes coaching, practice, surrendering, letting go of fear and being open to receive, to increase all levels of intuition!* I have found this to be consistently true which is why I have created a new focus of developing spiritually and intuitively for my training program. It is also why I have been so outspoken about my own experiences in this book.

Clearing the Self (Energetic Healing Part I)

Open the doors to new opportunities.

Share your heart. Be in the moment.
Surround yourself with Light and Love.

Go all the way. Don't hold back or hold within.
Beam all you are for others to experience.

Become fully what you are meant to be. Go further than you expect.

Go beyond the ordinary into the extra-ordinary.

Do not be afraid, you are not alone.

Healing Wounds (Energetic Healing Part II)

Balance between going forward and backward.

Care and comfort is what is needed to replenish the self.

Special friends will help you overcome obstacles.

Tell him you are sorry. Then embrace the light.

Be clear regarding what you want and go after it.

Lighten up in all you do and all you are.

Believe in the self fully.

Stay centered and aware to realize your dreams.

Find your truth and stay there.

Journey well my friend.

Why not release the hurt and go after what you want.

Believe me when I say forgive me. I am sorry too.

Tell him he needs to go on, so he can be free.

Heal the hurt and go forward.

Let go of expectations.

Changing Beliefs (Energetic Healing Part III)

Believe you can do it, and just do it!

Clear from the head that what hinders your path.

Send waves of love to all in need.
No longer carry the burdens of others passed down.

Take into the crown, Divine Light to show you the way.

Spread your wings and fly.

Clear out the soul, especially around the heart what no longer serves.

Allow light to trickle in and bless the aura.

Shake loose the ties that bind.

New Light is coming in to pave a new way.
Continue to get ready.

Allow Divine Light to shine on your face.

Be in the brilliance of the Light always.

Break loose the ties that bind. Be set free.

Healing Relationships Energetically (Energetic Healing Part IV)

I don't want you to go. Let's build our future.

Listen more fully with your whole being.

Soar with angels. Don't hold back!

Your feet are restless. You will be going to new places.

Bring sunlight into your life. Fill up the places that are dark.

Settle into the known and then shake the pieces to fully explore what other possibilities are.

Tell what is in your heart to others. Go forward and with full expression of what is important to you.

Live within the boundaries laid out and you will die within. Allow your Spirit to Soar!

Shake loose the ties that bind. Give up limitation.

Ease the pain, receive all that you need.

Breach no contracts.

Tell him what is on your mind, then release him.

Pick up the pieces of your life and become whole.

Glow with the times.

Sway and move to the music of your choice.

Let Light and Love be your healing motto.

Tell her I am sorry for some of the things I did in the past to hurt her.

Be careful who you love, that they honor and respect what is in your heart.

Open to new dimensions.

Stay under the umbrella of Light and Love when the going gets tough and you will be protected.

Reshaping Family Energy Patterns (Energetic Healing Part V)

Be frank about what needs to be said.

Create and set boundaries that will help.

Open the doors that bind.

Give windows to the self-imposed cylinder and take time to open when needed to allow light and love to come in.

Tell your truth to all those around you.

Let go of attachment to the outcome.

Call in the Light before, during, after the time you speak your truth to get clarity and be heard.

Patience. The fullness of Life comes when we trust in the Lord.

Share all you have for others to grow and heal.

Receive in return love and abundance.

Widen your dreams to include others in your heart.

178   **Development of the Healer**

RECEIVING GUIDANCE

Divine Intervention: Prayers for Protection

This section is a collection of instances of Divine Intervention that have happened to me over the years. I report them to alert the reader to take more time to connect with guidance and hear its message, because it can not only save your life, but save the life of those you love.

All the things that I have reported are true and happened to me. I never would have believed possible the things I am telling you. But it is time to tell these stories and not hold back. Once you learn it is possible to develop intuitive gifts, you will have additional encouragement to do what seems impossible. I always loved a challenge and I challenge you to connect more fully with your spiritual direction and watch how you life changes!

Mary Jo Bulbrook

Watch out Bill

The birth of my middle son Bill starts his Divine protection through my mother's influence. Before I left for the hospital mom prayed to the Sacred Heart of Jesus that all would go well and indeed it did. We are Catholic and that is the spiritual tradition I was raised in. The children grew leaps and bound over the years. I wondered how the time flew. How these tiny cells could grow into three handsome over six foot tall men was a miracle in itself. One day I received that dreaded phone call that all parents worry about. My son had been involved in an accident and was in the hospital.

I rushed to his side to find Bill in the emergency room and in pain from a broken jaw. I was told he and his friends left the high school at lunchtime and were horsing around in a parking lot. Bill was on the hood of one of his friend's car and the friend took off accidentally throwing him to the ground. As I entered the room I encountered a group of high schoolers very scared and sorry. Years later the told me the real story! He was operated on and a pin put in his jaw. I remember working on him in the recovery room by unruffling his energy field. Soon he was home and on the mend.

Two years later I was teaching in Florida. I awoke from a dream that Bill was going to be in another car accident! I began to worry and wondered if I should call him and tell him not to drive. I thought to myself, "It's a fat chance he will stop driving if I tell him not to drive. He will think I am crazy and ignore me!" It did seem ridiculous as I knew that was not the answer.

I relied on the old stand by—prayer. I asked for protection for my son. When Bill picked me up at the airport the next day I told him of the dream and asked that he be careful and pray. That evening while I was resting Bill came and asked me for the use of my car to go to work. He said that he had bad tires and didn't have the money to get them fixed. I said to buy the new tires and he could pay me when he got the money. I said that I wanted to go get a Christmas tree that night and would need my the station wagon. I then said, "Oh you take my car, I can get the tree when you come home."

That night when he came home he was all excited and said he had a near miss. He was pulling out from his job at Carolina Meadows when a woman came from around the bend speeding. He had to go into the ditch to keep her from hitting him! As he went into the ditch, he turned the wheel around and the car jumped with force back onto the highway with a thud. If he had been driving his own car with the bad tires, it might have been a different story!

Trip Over Wellington, NZ

One day as I was flying from Christchurch to Wellington several years ago, I realized I had not prayed for a safe journey. I took the time to pray to the angels and as I looked out the window I saw an angel underneath the wings of the airplane holding the plane up. I thought to myself, what a strange position for an angel to be in. We were going in for a landing at a very steep angle. All of the sudden, probably no more that 5 minutes after I prayed, we made a very steep ascent! In all of my years flying I have never experienced anything like that. A little while later the pilot came on and said in a controlled but calm way, "Sorry ladies and gentlemen, but we had to make a quick upward turn as we lost visibility suddenly. We would be circulating around and try again, not to worry." I looked out the window and saw an angel on *top* of the wings this time, and indeed I knew not to worry!

Near Miss: Donna on the Road

Donna Duff and I were working in our office together at the Point in Carrboro, NC about eight years ago. One night I left early to go home and she stayed behind as she was going to take a class in Greensboro, NC that evening, about a one hours trip away. As I walked to my car I heard a voice say, "You will never see Donna again." I stopped dead in my tracks and listened again. The voice repeated the message. I became scared and confused about what to do next. Should I go back and tell Donna not to go? What should I do? I went inside to get guidance and realized that the voice was not panicky but calm. I decided to pray to the angels to keep her safe and not go back and tell her not to go. I felt OK and continued walking to my car.

That night while I was reading, Donna came in late. I called from the other room asking who it was. She said she almost never made it. I jumped up from my chair and went to her. She said that while driving to Greensboro there was a car coming in her lane at her and would have hit her head on as there was a car next to her as well. She braced for the "hit" and suddenly the car next to her pulled off the road and the car heading toward them went between them. I told Donna about the premonition I had and we both thanked the angels for saving her life!

I remembered a story told to me by the director of the Rhine Institute in Durham, NC where J.B. Rhine, the famous psychic that started the first university-based laboratory on psychic phenomena. He told me one day when I was teaching at the Institute, that while he was manning the telephone lines one evening a woman called very distressed. She had dreamed of her husband being killed in a hunting accident. Since he had not planned to go hunting she dismissed the premonition. Then one day out of the clear blue sky he announced to her he was going hunting. She did not tell him of her dream and he was killed.

The woman was inconsolable and in anguish. It taught me especially after my experiences, that premonitions are given to us for a reason. Learn to trust what you get and work to be a clear channel. The best resource for the information you get is to pray. Go to a source higher than human nature and *pray for guidance*!

What I Thought Was Sky-Diving

In June, 1999 I was going to teach EH in Detroit for Kathy Sinnett. My business manager and son Bill announced to me that he was going skydiving that weekend. I wailed, "Oh no Bill, don't tell me that. I don't think I want to know!" We both laughed and I told him to be careful and that I loved him.

On the second day of teaching on Sunday we were having a late lunch. The group of us sitting together were having fun chatting about nothing at all when suddenly Bill appeared to me. I told the group that he was going sky diving the weekend and I was worried as a mother always is when her children do things that are dangerous. I asked the group if they would take a minute with me and pray for the safety of my son. We did in silence, each praying in our own way. Kathy Sinnett said, "Tell me when you get home what happened if anything!" I assured her that I would.

The next morning when I was home and Bill came to work I casually asked him how his weekend was. He told me he almost died. He said that he did not go sky diving but went white water rafting instead. He had been tossed out of the boat and at first he did not worry. He held onto his oar when he fell in so that he would not loose it. Unfortunately, he got trapped and held down by the oar that got jammed in some rocks. He realized that he better do something quick or he was going to die!

All of the sudden he was able to break free by pushing hard against the oar and it gave way. I told him of what my students and friends did in praying for him. The prayers were about the time of the near miss drowning. I said to him, "You have to remember to pray Bill. Don't just count on me and my friends to do it for you! *Develop a prayer life for yourself.*"

I am grateful to be able to teach my son this lesson in a way that he could really hear it and not be a lecturing mom. It is hard to pass on to our children information about spirituality. *Ask for guidance how to do it and then just do it for someday it may save your children's life or bring them comfort in time of need.* Spirituality is one of the best resources you can teach your children!

The Angels Turn Over the Car

My friend Eleanor and I were driving from Wellington across the North Island of New Zealand. It was a cold and wet rainy winter day in July. The rain turned to sleet and then to snow as the temperatures dropped. I watched the car in front of us start to skid and then go off the road and get ready to turn and come back on the road and in a position to hit me smack in the passengers door. (Remember in NZ they drive on the other side of the road.) I excitedly said, "They are out of control. They are going to hit us!" As we braced ourselves to be hit, the oncoming car turned over on its side. We stopped and ran back to the car. My friend had to craw up the underside of the car to open the door and free the trapped passengers. There was an elderly couple in the car. When the woman took off her seat belt she fell on top of her husband. We assisted them out of the car and in the mean time several others stopped to help. The woman was in shock. We took her to our car while the others who came to our rescue helped the gentleman out. My friend sat in the front seat with her arm around the trembling woman. I sat in the back seat and held her energy that was in spasm. As I held it for about five minutes I could feel it "snap" back into place. The woman began to sob and was finally calmed enough I could leave to check on her husband. He was walking around and did not appear injured.

When the police came, the group of people helped to turn the car right side up. The only damage to the car was a broken mirror on the outside of the car. The police determined that the couple was well enough to drive the short distance to their home. Eleanor and I got back into our car and followed the elderly couple to their home.

We went into their home, dried off, got a cup of tea, had a nice chat, and drove on to our workshop site. On reflecting what had happened after the crisis was over, I realized that the angels must have turned the car over to keep them from hitting me. I was not hurt, nor were they, nor was there damage to the car. What could have been a tragedy was prevented. There is no doubt in my mind about the power of connecting with angels!

P.S. I hope you enjoyed these five true stories about my experiences with Divine Intervention while I travelled to many places teaching HT and EH. I work with angels and with other spiritual beings that are based on my Catholic heritage. However, I am not suggesting for you to believe in what I believe in. I want to encourage you to work on you own spiritual path and those resources that offer you protection, guidance and comfort.

Mary Jo Bulbrook
Carrboro, North Carolina

Angels Light the Way

Just before the "angel craze" began, I was going through great change and expanding my creative process. Angel designs that were divinely inspired began drawing out on paper (in much the way that messages have been known to happen). Angels appeared to me as full sketches, in many designs. They would draw out for me, as I woke in the middle of the night, or at odd times of the day, even once as I talked on the phone with a friend! Ten, then fifteen to thirty, forty of them. Unlike other designing I had done before, these needed no corrections. In fact when I felt "I" could improve on them, I'd ruin something meant to be left as it was. I would then have to go back to the original sketch and use the one exactly as the angels gave it to me.

I had already had been creating resin-work jewelry pins so it seemed natural to reproduce these angel line designs and hand painted and finish them for people to wear or display showing their connection to angels. Thanks to the vision and encouragement of my mentor, Mary Jo Bulbrook, I went full out to produce and make available these creations in order to spread angel light. Mary Jo and I both know it is our contribution to foster angel energy in this time of need in our troubled world. So what began previous to all of the above—angel statues in my home collected from travels while teaching Healing Touch or as gifts from family and friends—has evolved into an angel-design business that continues to this day. Then something happened.

One day one of the angels identified with an actual person. The first came as a flash of insight from a sketch drawn out during a workshop in Colorado. A member of our sharing group named Sally spoke, my pen doodled water waves, then a tiny conch shell and a finger that shaped itself into a mermaid angel lounging on a rock as waves curled over her. Intrigued and in awe of this, I felt compelled to give this as a message to Sally who with hand-to-heart revealed the angelic identification to us both, "I absolutely live by the water," she declared. "I head for the ocean whenever I feel distressed, alone or in need. It's my spiritual connection. Nothing soothes me more!"

"Well," I said. "This angel has a message: 'The conch shell is offered to you because you listen so well to others.'" She and I hugged each over and over as we shared this experience. This message was the first of many the angels revealed to me.

The founder of the holistic nurses association that sponsored our holistic healing group at that time was seriously ill. Many hundreds of us were in prayer vigils around the world for her. I had the strong urge to send one of my angel pins for her pillow. This was "Elegant Angel," her specific angelic connection.

I created another design for a friend, Elloree, called "Imperial Angel" which came to me with information of a life she'd experience in an oriental setting that she knew was absolutely correct for her. For my daughter-in-law there was "Delicious Angel." For one whose last name was Bell, there was the "Angel Bell" design. An engineer friend of amazon proportions and I were flabbergasted at "Wonder Angel" that appeared for her. "I used to dress as Wonder Woman for Halloween," she said.

But the most incredible identification was "Moon Cherub." In Richmond, Virginia, the coordinator of our workshop emphasized, "You must meet Ruth who will be attending today. She gets Angel letters" (material from angels). On meeting her I found this sweet person also dedicated to angel energy. When she told me how her five year old daughter Amanda had passed away a year before with leukemia, I felt a signal of an angel communication. "Ruth," I said. "I feel that one of my angel pins shows an angel identification with your daughter." And I thought immediately of a cherub, but which one? There were two, one with a moon. I told her, "It's a cherub." Ruth looked into my eyes and said, "That's wonderful!" She showed me Amanda's picture—a cherub if there ever was one! Amazed I saw a whistle come out of Amanda's lips!

"Did she whistle?" I asked. "She loved to whistle," Ruth replied. "And I have to tell you I feel led to show you this latest Angel Letter." And as she did, I saw the words "Moon Daughter" and knew that it was the "Moon Cherub" angel for Amanda. "My daughter was a moon daughter," Ruth grinned when I told her. "Often when she was in pain and it wouldn't let her sleep, Amanda would beg me to bring her to see the moon. I'd wrap her up and we'd go into the yard where she could watch the moon and fall asleep." When Ruth mentioned that her daughter had seemed like an "old soul," I felt the truth of it. She said Amanda at five years old had picked out her own grave site in a rural cemetery in their hometown and asked that a stone bench be put there for people to sit and meditate. Ruth feels that people will be enlightened spiritually as they meditate there.

Amanda was the first child identification with one of my angel motifs, but not the last. Of the more than 60 designs that have surfaced, the most recent is for Lydia Xuan, an adopted baby from China now living in middle Georgia, USA. Hers is Manchurian Angel and she truly is just that. I have truly been inspired, that indeed, Angels Light the Way!

Anne Boyd
Augusta, Georgia

The Story Behind Angelight

Several years ago, Anne Boyd and I were in teacher training for Healing Touch together in Georgia. At the break we were walking down the street with the class on the way to lunch. At this meeting Anne had shared the new angel pins she had created from divine inspiration. As I held them in my hand and felt the energy from them, I said to her, "You really need to do something with these angels. They are very special! And, you need to change the name of your business to reflect what you have created."

On the walk we started to brainstorm a new name for the angel focused business. Each of us put forth different names and felt the energy of each name to see how it "felt energetically!" After several minutes out of my mouth came Angelight. We both stopped in the street, looked at each other and simultaneously said, "Yes." Angelight became the new name and a new business was born out of our mutual connection to angels.

Together we picked the logo angel for the business and she was named Angelight. One day I was preparing to help Anne market angel energy by creating angel T-shirts to wear at our conferences.

Bill, my middle son, asked me what I was doing. I told him my intent and he thought that was a great idea! I was surprised that a teenager would want to wear a T-shirt with an angel on it but pleased that he felt comfortable connecting with angels. I was trying to create a motto for the shirt. Bill and I finally settled on, "Angels light the way. Ask and you shall receive." I left to go to my office and see a friend who was coming for a treatment that day. When she came in, I showed her the new T-shirt and asked her what she thought. She liked it very much. I then showed her the saying I was going to put on the back. She looked at it and thought for a moment. She said, "You really don't need the ending, just use, "Angels light the way." I knew she was right. I felt a little uncomfortable with the second part because I could hear others saying: "I asked and they didn't come." Many are unaware just how angels come in our life. They always come, however, we may be too focused in a certain outcome we may not notice when they help us. That was the birth of Angelight, and Angels light the way. It can be said as a statement or as a prayer for help. It works either way!

One of the most important stories for me about Anne's angels involves my caring for a woman through my volunteer work in Hospice. She was dying of metastatic brain cancer and was hospitalized very sick. When I walked into the room she was all curled up in a fetal position and very, very sick. I approached her to talk and she looked up startled very much in discomfort. I realized that something was very wrong with her field. I stepped back and quietly worked to find the edge of her aura. What I found was a very jagged edge, hyperextended at the head and close at the edge of her body. I unruffled the top edge in and the bottom out. After I did this she visibly relaxed and opened her eyes. I walked over to the bed and showed her the angel pins I had in a box that I was taking to a workshop the next day. I asked if she would like one. She opened the box and handled them very gently. The energy of the angel went into her and I saw a marked difference with each angel she picked up. She told me she wanted to find the right one. So she picked up about 10 angels and repeated the same process. Each handling of the angels brought greater strength and vitality to her field. She finally selected one and we pinned it on her. I left and promised to return the next day.

When I returned the next day, she was sitting up in bed playing cards with her husband! I was absolutely astounded at the changes in her. To me it was as if the energy came into her from each of the angels. I will never know what made the changes, but she went home shortly and lived several months and got to experience the love of her young children and family once again. In the end, does it really matter what made the difference? I am betting on the angels because I have experienced their power first hand and know there is a force there like none other. I know that I can count on the angels to light the way!

Mary Jo Bulbrook
Carrboro, North Carolina

Angelic Inspirations

The following are from the Angelic Inspiration cards that came from readings in the EH classes. I am including them here related to the section on Divine Guidance Stories. I am very committed to encourage people to connect with angels as I have seen the power in my own life and want to share that with others.

The front of the brochure describing my business has the Energetic Healing Angel on the front of it. The story behind that angel is very incredible and I would like to share it now.

A number of years ago I approached Anne Boyd, CHTP/I to create an angel for me to use with my work in Healing Touch. At the time, Anne, through guidance, channeled some wonderful angels that she made up into angel pins to focus one's energy with angelic presencing. I have witnessed the power of these angels over time.

I commissioned Anne to do a special angel design for a T-shirt to share angel energy for all that would see it. Although Anne sent me the picture, for some reason unknown to me at that time we did not get around to using that angel. In the meantime though Anne changed the angel for some reason and made a pin from that change.

Then in 1997 when I brought healers from Australia, New Zealand and South Africa to the USA to give workshops all over the country I decided that I needed to have a new angel for what I was currently doing. I asked her permission to use the angel for the Energetic Healing Program because of my emphasis on the spiritual aspects of healing. She told me she would be honored to have me use the angel and this angel known as Energetic Healing Angel.

I had commissioned another artist to put this angel on a van I bought to travel around with the tour group. The artist told me that when he was working on it in the parking lot, many would come by and look at the angel. He was very surprised at their reaction. In preparation for the trip I called Anne to send me a copy of the Angel so that I could also make a T-shirt with Energetic Healing Angel on it. In the meantime, I found the original angel that Anne had sent me years ago. The day I was working on the final phase of organizing the T-shirt there were three of us in my kitchen looking over the current version of the angel.

Anne joined us for the tour. I went up to her excitedly and asked how she liked the angel on the side of the van. She shook here head and walked away. Disappointed and confused, I ran after her and asked what was wrong. She shook her head again and said, "You changed my angel. I can't believe that you would change my angel." She walked away. I became very distress and wondered what had happened. I knew that the graphic artist did not change the angel. Finally I realized that the angel I used was the original one Anne had sent me, not the changed one she did later! I ran after her and said, "Guess what Anne? I didn't change the angel, you did!"

I related the story to her. She smiled and said, "The angel didn't want to be changed! She stayed in hiding, until it was ready for her to come and be connected with the EH program and the progress of my work to that time. Just when you think you are in charge of your life, notice how Spirit has stepped in and guided you to another path! I am very pleased and proud to have the EH angel shine her Light to come when you call, when you are in need and forget to ask. This is what she has to offer and more!"

The message on the front of the T-shirt says:

> I come when you call.
> I await your tuning in.
>
> I listen to your heart
> And come
> When you are in need
> And forget to ask.
>
> This is what I have to offer
> and more.

—Spiritual Guidance

This message came to me when I was treating a university professor. I shared the message with her and got her permission to use the reading as a description of my philosophy in my work — that is, helping people to connect with spirit.

Below are some of the inspirational messages. Notice which ones you can identify with or that resonate to you. Then meditate on the message and observe the changes in your energy system.

Resonate to the sounds and sights of the earth.

Light and love surrounds you.

Be still and receive the Light.

Be kind to those who are difficult.

Develop a lifestyle of healing in all that you do and all that you are.

The path before you is at you feet. Feel the earth's vibration to help you heal.

Light the way for others to see.

You have gone beyond the individual path to the collective.

Divine will vs. your will.

Experience your joy and offer it back to others.

Be open. The levels beyond are trying to reach you.

Your highest good is in our hands. We are with you.

Beyond the horizon is your life's path.

Find your truth and heart space by connecting more fully with us.

Mary Jo Bulbrook
Carrboro, North Carolina

CONNECTING WITH MARY

Meeting Mary

In April, 1999 I attended a HT Level IIA class at St. Mary's Medical Center in Knoxville, TN. The first night we learned to do the Chakra Spread in a chair. As I kneeled on the ground to work on the lower part of the JB's body, I felt and saw the presence of Mother Mary. It was not at all what one would expect (dramatic, flash of light, etc.) but instead she stood there as a quiet presence of love and compassion. She gave me a verbal message for JB (private), then told me: "Show her how to let go, help her to let go." Then a profound non-verbal understanding passed between Mary and I: she was there for JB, and also for me, for guidance, support, healing, and love. I continued with the Chakra Spread, humbled, but unawed by the experience. At the time it seemed perfectly normal and natural for Mary to be there. I always ask for and receive guidance when doing healing work, but this was clearly different. At the same time my left-brain was searching for a way to explain this experience: "Well, of course Mary is here, it *is* St. Mary's Hospital after all."

After the session I asked JB about her religious background before sharing the vision/message. It turns out that she was Methodist, open to spiritual things, but not a regular church-goer. When I shared the message from Mary with her, JB began to cry and told me about some recent family turmoil with her daughter. Since JB was quite emotional and the message/experience seemed very private, I left it up to her as to whether to share any of this with the class. She decided to do so and also recalled that many years ago she was born in that hospital, but had not been to Knoxville in quite a long time.

Later that night I called my wife Kathleen and told her about the experience. Since she grew up in a Catholic family (I did not), I asked her for the words to the "Hail Mary Prayer." Even though I had no prior connection with Mary, I have used that prayer for personal devotion often since that time. During the rest of the HT workshop I visited the hospital chapel (it held a beautiful statue of Mary) for prayer and guidance as well.

Later that weekend I was working with another workshop participant, DW. When the class gathered together to talk about the recent healing session, she shared that while I was working on her the only thing she remembered was a very distinct and powerful scent of roses. When she said this I was a little disappointed because I thought that I (ego talking here) had done some powerful work on her and all she could report was the smell of flowers! The instructor asked DW if this meant anything to her. She reported no associations other than it being very pleasant. The instructor then commented that it was interesting that the smell of roses occurred while I was working on DW since the appearance or fragrance of roses is often associated with the presence of Mary.

These experiences were both humbling and empowering for me. I used to see reports on TV of sightings and messages from Mary and skeptically dismissed these kind of stories as the product of overzealous piety or well meaning wish fulfillment. The need to judge others, about their religious sincerity or anything at all, is just one thing Mary has help me learn to let go.

To see Mary and stand in the light of such overwhelming compassion and love, even for a just few moments, makes me want to live in that space all the time. My work with energy-based healing has helped me work towards that goal, both in giving and receiving. The more we seek to help and heal others, the more we are helped and healed ourselves.

Dan Trollinger
Durham, North Carolina

Conversations with Mary

Author's Note: While preparing this section I ran into many obstacles. I finally let go of my frustration and listened to guidance. I realized that I was being called to relate my experience with Barbara and her story from her book *Conversations with Mary*.

Through a mutual HT colleague in Florida, who is also a link to the work with the Indigenous people talked about later on in the book, Barbara contacted me to see if I would be interested in her book about Mary. I had a chance to read the book and think about Barbara's experiences with the Virgin Mary during my trip to Australia this summer. Our journey's paralleled each other in a number of ways. While working on this book, I realized that I had not thanked her and told her how much I enjoyed her book. When I did this I also told her about my book on Healing Stories and asked if she had a story to submit. She offered a chapter from her book. Barbara's gift of sharing her story of her encounter with Mary encouraged me to share my "Mary stories" with others. Then when I found out that Dan, the editor for this book, also had experiences with Mary, I knew Mary had a hand in helping to produce this book. I felt she connected us together to pass on the word of how Mary is available to those who are open to receive, even those ordinary folks like us, who are not looking for it. Trust the process and be open.

True spiritual guidance is quite different from ego based, controlled experience. The open heart attracts others of like mind. Enjoy this brief excerpt from Barbara's book and I also invite you to hear her whole story about *Conversations with Mary*.

Our Lady of Clearwater, 1996

"Dear Mother Mary," I prayed fervently. "Will you protect me if I publish my stories?"

Her reassuring reply: "Don't be afraid, my child. Tell your stories."

"Please send me a sign," I pleaded. "It has been more than thirteen years since you appeared to me. Won't you please come again?"

Just a few days later I was astonished to hear the words of the announcer on the evening news.

"Scientists are still searching for an earthly explanation for the forty-foot-tall image resembling the Madonna that has appeared on nine sections of a smoked glass window in the Seminole Finance Building on December 17th," the television newscaster reported, with amazement clear in his tone.

I stood in the family room and watched, stunned, as television cameras swept over the thousands of visitors gathered that evening. I remembered that it had been just a few days earlier that I had asked Mother Mary for a sign. Steady, I thought. Don't let your imagination run away with you. I stood, motionless as if glued to the spot.

"The infirm, the faithful, and the hopeful have all come to Clearwater, Florida, this week before Christmas." The reported continued. "The Associated Press has reported that almost half a million people have flocked to see an image on a financial building said to resemble the Madonna. The building's owner has no explanation for the Virgin Vision, but he acknowledges that an incredible artist and divine intervention must have played a part in creating this glorious image of the Virgin Mary."

Hearing this broadcast took my breath away. My hands began to tremble and my heartbeats quicken. My husband and I were planning to have our annual Christmas Day dinner with my son, Erick, and his family in Palm Harbor, just a few short miles form the Clearwater building. Was this a divine coincidence?

I believe what Carl Jung taught: There are no accidents. He described a phenomenon called synchronicity. It occurs when two simultaneous events that we call coincidences are related in a profound way that is not casual. These events command our attention or may even change our life. For me, the image in Clearwater was a synchronous event. Could this image of the Mother Mary be a demonstration for me? I wondered.

On Christmas Day we drove along US 19 toward the finance building. At first, the city streets seemed normal. Then suddenly the traffic slowed to a crawl as we approached the building. As we inched forward, I lowered the car window to see if I could see the building or the window. I saw nothing. Then the pace quickened.

Adrenaline surged through me as a traffic cop stopped our car to allow streams of people to cross the highway. He grinned at us through the windshield, and my husband rolled down his window.

"Merry Christmas," Chip called. "Quite a crowd, hey?"

"It's unbelievable," the young officer said, laughing. "We're expecting twenty-five thousand people here today."

For days the newscasters had been treating the vision lightly, but not one scientist had yet been able to explain the formation of this heavenly shape. All around me, reverently silent children and adults knelt on the asphalt. Some made the sign of the cross over their tattered T-shirts or exquisite holiday finery. Most people clasped rosary beads in hopeful hands. I became extremely aware that I was not a Roman Catholic and also acutely aware of the importance of Mary in the lives of others. Then the thought came to me that I did not have to be Catholic to honor Mary as the Universal Mother.

The melodious sounds of Spanish, French, and Italian blended beautifully with the crisp New England and soft Southern Accents. Metal wheelchairs and wooden crutches intermingled with exquisite emeralds and dazzling diamonds. No one seemed conscious of status or apparel. We were the people of faith and hope, all coming together this Christmas Day in this spiritual moment—all believing in the unseen side of life. We are all one.

I peered ahead to a makeshift altar where candles of all colors and shapes flickered dimly in the bright sunlight. Nearby, on a drab, gray concrete wall in front of the windows, an ordinary, small cardboard box held donations for All Children's Hospital in St. Petersburg, Florida. Single roses, pink and red, and small bouquets of brightly colored flowers, some plastic, were scattered on the wall. A red poinsettia or two were casually placed on the ground.

The holiness and reverence of the moment were palpable in the air. Continuing to look up at the image and expecting to be unimpressed, I was stunned by my reaction. My breath was momentarily taken away, my heart began to beat rapidly, and the hair on my arms stood up straight. A large chill ran up my spine, as I stood transfixed. I consciously centered myself and took some deep breaths. Now don't get carried away, my objective self said. Look at this rationally.

Suddenly, I heard Mother Mary's nurturing voice reverberating in my heart. It was as if a tape recorder had been turned on. The clarity and sweetness of the sound took me by surprise.

"It has been said that I would come and give messages to the planet," she said. "I have come to Clearwater, Florida, because the name of the city is significant. This is an important part of my message. You must have clear water. The pollution of the water must stop. This is not an option. This is necessary for the survival of the planet. The seas and the oceans are your lifeline."

"It is no coincidence that you are here this day," the blessed voice continued. "I have chosen you as a vehicle through whom my message will be spread. For many months you have been debating whether to accept this assignment. This is my last call to you. You must tell of this day and of our previous meetings in a book."

In that sacred moment, my heart overflowed with love. My eyes, brimmed full with tears. Unashamed, I let them fall freely. Deeply moved, I looked up at the Blessed Mother and silently said, "Oh, Mary, I don't know whether I have the courage to tell of our hallowed meetings, I am so afraid of ridicule."

"Yes, tell your stories," she lovingly urged. "Let it be known unto all the people, for they are stories about the sacredness of all life. This is not a question of religion. Those are man-made—it is a question of faith and souls being denied access to the body. All individuals must be responsible for their actions. To do otherwise is to create havoc on the earth. You must tell of the miracles of birth and the choice of adoption. This is my message to you: Put forth your book for all whose eyes are open to see."

(Afterward) The rainbow image of the Virgin Mary that appeared on December 17, 1996 on a financial building has not faded. The site at Drew Street and Route 19 in Clearwater, Florida has been leased to a Catholic group from Ohio. And so my prayer that his site would evolve into an international shrine for people of all faiths is unfolding. A chain-link fence now encloses the blacktop parking lot and chairs welcome visitors. Brightly colored flowers have been planted and a wooden kneeling bench has been provided by one of the faithful. The hundreds of notes, the rosary beads, the candles and other mementos that were left on the concrete wall have disappeared. A sign politely asks the public not to leave anything behind.

But the public does leave something behind that cannot be measured by science nor seen by the skeptic. The now more than one million visitors leave behind their Courage, their Love, and their Faith in the unseen side of life and they take away Hope, Peace and Strength. Theses are qualities not available at any price. There remains a comfort and a splendor in this scientifically unexplained vision. The important facts are these. The lovely image of the Madonna remains—it resonates with the faithful—and it is glorious!

Barbara Harris
Osprey, Florida

Prayers Are Cumulative

After receiving an e-mail that a mutual acquaintance had passed on, I knew I had to pray for her. As I sat in meditation saying the Rosary I saw N lying on a small infirmary cot with her Helper Being attending to her. As I said each "Hail Mary" the energy of the prayer entered her being in waves. She was in shock. First she was here on earth going about her life and the next thing she knew she was on the other side. The next day I repeated prayed again. She was still lying on the infirmary cot with her Helper Being sitting beside her. About half way through the Rosary, the Helper Being jumps up and says, "That's enough, there are so many prayers coming in, that's enough." I continued to pray. Now the energy of the prayers were neatly folded like a blanket and placed on a shelf to be used as needed. The third day of prayer found N sitting on her cot with her suitcases packed beside her. She was ready to enter the Light. Prayers *are* cumulative!

Cathy Mack
Garner, North Carolina

MESSAGES FROM MARY

Following are messages that I humbly received from Mary starting in 1993. I am pleased to share what she has given me, for it may help and guide you in your spiritual development as it has helped me. The messages were all recorded verbatim as they were given. However, I added the titles later.

Ten Tasks in Life

Awakened from a deep sleep, I saw an angel, like the one I saw at 12:15 a.m. when I went to bed. I thought that the angel wanted to give me information. As I arose and went into the living room to record the message, I heard a woman's voice and soon came to realize the message was from Mary, the mother of Jesus.

Dear one,
My heart reaches out to your heart,
Feeling all your feelings,
Experiencing all your experiences.

We are one in the Spirit,
The Unity of God made man –
My Son the Savior of the world.

Lighten up.
Be light in all that you do.
Care with the whole range of your being.

Experience the heart beat resonating deep within the soul.
Feel the presence of God surround you
As you surrender to the Divine Will.

The plan of God is to infuse the world with love
To counteract all of the negativity
That befalls alignment with darkness.

All that is beautiful
Will be yours
As you merge your will with God's.

This is a simple
Yet profound act of complete love
And obedience to the Holy will.

The fathoms are deep of buried pain within you and within others.
Healing needs to take place,
Releasing these buried places of restriction and confinement through
fear, rage, hurt, and resentment.

Anxiety that is free floating and hidden, robs the self of joy,
Creating an aimless skeleton of a being devoid of life giving
properties of joy, peace, and radiance.

The tasks are simple.

1) Open the being to the flood gates which house boundless joy. A
   simple act of trust in God and obedience to Divine will.

2) Honor the self first. Be committed to your family, the care takers
   and caretaking charges of yours, then embrace your friends in
   love, as well as your enemies as it is love that will transform the
   world.

3) Be reverent to all aspects of the earth, the air, water, land, plants,
   minerals and animals. All of these are God's creatures desirous
   of fulfilling their destiny which is service to God through
   interdependence of all creatures of the Holy One.

4) Make wise use of resources, personal and those of the earth.
   Align your will with the Spirit to "know" what is right.

5) Have right intention; be the best you can be at any moment in
   time, always striving to do and be better as you become more
   God-like.

6) Be patient and tolerant with the self and others. Differences are
   to be respected at all times being clear in one's path and not
   forcing that on another. Your modeling of you, your holiness,
   your achievements while living that holiness will be what will
   win others over who choose paths of lower spiritual attainment.

7)   There are many religious/spiritual paths that will lead you to oneness with God. Be tolerant and respectful of the path chosen not like you, as the inner light within a person is to be the guide.

8)   Know your truth by living your truth. Do not judge yourself nor others. Only follow your internal guidance sparkled with the Light of radiant beings who speak and live truth.

9)   Pray, fast (do without), sacrifice—give up ways and things you are shown to be of lesser alignment with wholeness and holiness.

10) Share God's truth by your beingness. Take each moment of the day to be your prayer, your offering to make this world a better place, for in doing so, the "whole" will be changed. Peace starts at home – in your heart, in your being – with those you love and those who are hard to love. Once this truth is realized this age will be transformed into a new golden age with less pain and suffering. Service is the tool to salvation of the self and the world. Align your will, life, and love with God's. That is all you need.

Pray to me and the other saints for guidance on the path. We readily await your attunement to our energies as we are eager to instruct.

Let go of things that don't make sense with the rational mind at times, for the new leader in the world is the feminine, the intuitive, not the male, the rational. That is not to say to abandon rationality, only to use it to operationalize intuition. Spiritually led choices are one in the unity of the Holy Spirit, God made man/woman.

Women power is in full force. The angels will show the way.

I go now but will return to you again in slumber for more messages for the world. Record these and soon you will be guided how to distribute the word passed to and through you from many sources.

Lovingly, Mary

Recorded by Mary Jo Bulbrook (1/8/93)

Leading One's Life

Your guardian angel who came last night visibly and this morning is the one charged with your journey. Pray to her as she is very powerful indeed and eager to serve you in your life's work.

Let go of petty differences and embrace your life in and with love. All is well, you are well, and the world is well. I go now but will return to you again in slumber for more messages for the world. Record these and soon you will be guided how to distribute the word passed to and through you from many sources.

Indeed you are to be a scribe for Divine Light. Be aware of that charge. Let go of your pain around your pervious earthly titles of Professor, etc. They are nothing compared to being a servant of God/Goddess. They are really one and the same, for it is the two God/Goddess which is the Divine One, the Ultimate. Goddess energy is the rule in this generation now and in the future rounding out the Divine Plan to Nirvana.

Guidance to you will be an internal knowing. Know that with every part of your being. Trust that. When things don't make rational sense that is OK. You will be led through any obstacle. The full scope of the intent may be closed to knowing at times but once the lesson is learned, the full awareness will be made known at some level.

Trust your being. Trust the beingness of others. Focus on the light and you will be well guided, guarded and grounded to accomplishing Divine will fulfilling the ultimate meaning of life.

I go now. Rest in peace. Return to your slumber.

Lovingly, Mary

P.S. I packed the angel card of faith after the session.

Recorded by Mary Jo Bulbrook (1/15/93)

Return to God
Dear one,

Harken to the sound of the angels who call you to the Almighty—the One in Christ. Favor returns to the earth as it tunes its frequency once again to God—away from darkness.

The plight of the world is one of internal and external balance—alignment/attunement with the forces of nature and with spiritual causes/effects to the tune of heavenly hosts which orchestrate the chant which realigns the being into spiritual centeredness with God forcing balance to return to one's life.

1) Find you center by being your center. Strengthen the weak spots in you by offering them up to God/Goddess forcing them to be sanctified and infused with light to show the way in darkness.

2) Pierce the darkness with joy. Find moment to moment joy in the task of daily living forcing the self to reevaluate the purpose of this destiny and meaning of each daily event/activity.

3) Center each day. Pray to the Lord, my father/son/mother/daughter. Seek comfort in the knowing of your intent to excel in the power of truth, justice, love and light.

4) Rest daily at deep levels. Renew the self frequently to reset the boundaries that have become off balance.

5) Right wrongs. Listen with your being, your essence, then follow the path.

6) Challenge your fears, lack of self esteem, hesitancy, resistance, laziness, overwork.

7) Call forth peace, love, justice to reset the world and individual balance. Those who choose to do this will change themselves and the world. Believe this and once again—the red sea will part—you will be safe from the enemy—darkness.

8) Challenge yourself to go further than today, yesterday. May your tomorrow be set with a firm, steady vision of these principles laid out.

9) Do not waver from your belief. When you become weak, ask for strength and you will be carried in the arms of God/Goddess, the ultimate one. I am the messenger of Divine Light to show you the way. Believe in me. Strengthen yourself by your beliefs. Let go of your doubts. Trust. Love. Sense the Goodness in all. Cling to that. Honor that strength and call it forth.

Go in peace. Return to slumber

Lovingly, Mary

(I saw Mary leave surrounded by a group. I heard Mary of Guadalupe and saw energy flowing from her hands.)

Recorded by Mary Jo Bulbrook (3/13/93)

Come to Me

Dear ones,

I come in haste to you tonight as the time is getting shorter to the impending disasters in the world.

1) Hold your ground. Be your ground. Stand firm in all you believe and need for your life's purpose to be complete. My outstretched hands are a symbol of a "centered" loving surrender to Divine Will, not submission nor of a servant quality, but a loving centeredness, capable of providing you and others with serenity. Unrest in the world, hurtful deeds come from misguided greed and reliance on earthly pleasures to satisfy every desire. This hedonistic approach to life allows the soul to be susceptible to unwanted influences that get us off the path.

2) Come to my bosom for replenishment. Pray to me and the other saints who desire to make contact with you in times of trial and trouble. The spirit world offers a multidimensional collection of untapped expertise in a variety of areas. We see and live where your vision ends. The scope of our world is to be an interface with earthly grounded individuals sensitive to receive and honor the word of God made man/woman through the medium of human capacity.

3) Love your neighbor and do not covet the possessions of others be they person, place or thing including emotional, spiritual, mental, or physical strength.

4) Honor you—all you are, all you have been, all you will become. Vow to rid the self of unwanted deeds that have hurt others deeply and not so deeply. You need only pause and I will come. I leave my scent the rose as my calling card for those unable to access any tangible connection to my soul from yours.

5) Be aware of all there is to be and fear nothing. God watches those who surrender to a Higher Power, a Divine calling of sound parenting.

Mother/father hear my plea. Love your children.
Touch their souls deeply to help them grow on their path.
Accept their limitations with loving kindness as they do deeds unworthy of their upbringing.

Trust their souls needed to be shaken and was within their own destiny. Being caught occurred because the demands of justice are to be realized on this earth to purify their misguided preoccupation with earthly things.

The Holy Spirit, the Divine One will center each of you through trials of all kinds. Call forth to us to help you. Center. Stabilize and be renewed in holiness, peace and serenity. Do not be bewildered by what you cannot understand. This process requires an act of faith, a leap to a perspective worthy of your awareness and pondering.

6) Keep open to the Divine light and stability, peace will return in time.

7) Be careful to replenish the soul daily as that is your only true substance of life.

I go now to return later.

Lovingly, Mary

Recorded by Mary Jo Bulbrook (3/93)

Embrace the Light

Dear one,

It is time to recognize what is about to happen. You are expected to assist in a very profound thing that is to take place. There are very many spirits that are aiding in what is about to happen. Do not be afraid to move forward and touch deeply the lives you are becoming intimately connected to, for you are the connector to their source. I have been aware of your reluctance to embrace the Light and all that is in store for you and others.

I have these messages for you today:

1) Be tolerant of all that is different from who and what you are and believe in. Each person, or aspect of life that is different is resonating to the Divine in the way that is most appreciative of what is needed for that person's soul development at that time. We are all meant to coexist in time and space together and be part of the life giving force of all aspects of life. You can choose the specifics of life, but know that there is a another way of doing things that best suits the life and awareness of those aspects of differentness.

2) Be helpful to everyone on their journey, supporting their steps each part of the way and helping them to believe in themselves, all that they stand for and embrace the Light. The Light is not for just one race, for one culture. The Light is the unifying force available to all people regardless of race, culture or believe. Step up the awareness of others to open to the Divine and approach Godliness which is important resource in the conduct of one's life. There will soon be available an intense learning for people to become more whole and holy and able to reach multidimensions of reality easily. The gifts that you have developed will aid you in helping others to develop their gifts. Know that I am with you in all things that you do and that you are. There will be no wanting for you in any way as the full opportunities are soon to come to you completely to realize the opportunities of the soul and its enfoldment.

3) Be kind to yourself in all aspects of life and know that there is no compromise when it comes to learning, loving, and living the truth.

4) Be friendly to the various forms of life. Treat each aspect with the graciousness and awareness that is befitting one who has reached Divine attunement.

5) Be Light in all that you do and that you are.

6) Be come a model of peacefulness and peaceful living between and among all aspect of life. You shall not want. Share the gifts that you have received and become childlike in the acceptance of the joys of life entering you and aiding in the process of the divine likeness of God.

7) Be of great fortitude in accomplishing what is needed and expected of you. That means caring for the self in such a way as to keep track of all that is good and divine within and without and embraces the Light, for there is no greater service that which serves the Divine. Do not fear, nor be reluctant to enter into deep relationships in all that you encounter. Each relationship has a deeper relationship waiting to be discovered therefore there is no need to cling onto the present or the past. Be more open to other opportunities that will be forthcoming. We will help you to discover the power in the relationships and become all that is needed to enter into them without destroying the structure of you live. Find the forgiveness deep into your heart and there will be no doubting what is possible.

I go now to return later. Please become awakened. Much is lost because of your reluctance to awaken and become informed. We will help you to center in all that you do and all that you are. Find the peacefulness through nature and you will not suffer.

Lovingly, Mary

Recorded by Mary Jo Bulbrook (3/11/93, Auckland, NZ)

Break Free from Limitation

I see before me much trial and tribulation for the world. Suffering is/
has come because of the limitations placed on those who fear and
jealousy has become a way of life. Return to the safety of God's
eternal peace of the soul resting in the chamber of the heart, ready to
burst forward bringing a sense of knowing/direction for ones life.
The branches of religions are just that. One in the Lord manifested
in different directions reaching beyond into a vast array of scary
patterns that depend on desperation to keep them in place.

1) Break free from limitation. Soar with the angels.

2) Write your internal song longing to be sung.

3) Open the door to sanctified living by associating with those
things/experiences of the Divine.

4) Honor the earth.

5) Kiss the core with Divine Love ridding the erosion caused by
greed, carelessness behaviors that are selfish to say and deserv-
ing of little energy to maintain the unhealthy pattern.

6) Breech no promises made in haste that are from the heart.

7) Unlock the secrets bound up in your being and fulfill your hope
and longing for full expression of your heart's desire.

8) Count on me. Come to me. Establish your base of operation from
and in me. Linger no more in the stuck place. Come full circle to the
hearts delight. Regain your peacefulness by being your peacefulness. Enrich the rageful energy by a lattice work of love that can break
up the particles to be dissolved into the essence of life and loving
gestures of kindness to soften the hardest of hearts and the gravest
of stuck emotions that have eroded their current state of being.

9) Free the soul. Free the being. Become who you were meant to be
by embracing love. Soar with all people the entire place of live and
live as the base of operation of all time and eternity will be yours.

Return to slumber. I go now.

Lovingly, Mary

Recorded by Mary Jo Bulbrook (6/93)

Sexual Expression in the World
Dear one,

Thank you for awakening to receive messages today.
I am concerned about sexual expression in the world.
It is not OK to exploit the body or others in any way.

My message for today is as follows:

Be kind to the self and support all aspects of the individual that needs nurturance and self-expression.

It is tolerant to stimulate the self in ways that enhance the Divine Light and serves the purpose of the soul.

Only that which serves this purpose is to be expressed.
At times it is difficult to know that this is or how to do it.
I will instruct you in the correct procedure.

Love and fulfill the full expression as it emerges, not through force or outside stimulation. The gentle flowing from one aspect of the self to the other will occur naturally and be very fulfilling. Follow the peaks and valleys of attunement to the Divine and awaken all of the senses to their full expression. This process occurs naturally and flows easily. The stopping and starting without the loving expression distorts and masks the true nature of sexuality which is an outgrowth of loving from the heart, not from the genitals or from lust or manipulation of a another just to satisfy a need of yours.

Keep in grace and allow sexuality to come naturally. You will be rewarded for keeping this commandment I request of you at this point in your life. Be patient and this too will become a beautiful point in your life. I go now. Thanks for listening.

Lovingly, Mary

Recorded by Mary Jo Bulbrook (3/12/94, Christchurch, NZ)

Reflection

Dear one,

Thank you for responding to my request to receive messages from me. Tonight it seems that is it appropriate that you reflect on all that has happened to you and realize that when I first came to you that you doubted the authenticity of the messages. I think by now from all of the experiences that you have had it is time to believe in what you do and what you are. There has come the time to repeat often the reflection of the God within and all that symbolizes, namely peace, joy, love and truth.

Reflect on all that you are, where you have come from and where you are going. Become clearer you though it was going to be. Take more time to reflect and receive direction from her spiritual guides and teachers. Books are to become the language of love, to show the world a new way, a way how to transcend language and expression that will repeat the necessary components of faith, hope, love, and charity.

There is no opportunity like the present to renew the kinship ties that have served generations well. The ancient ones are now longing to have a clearer connection with you and you are to return to your spiritual roots.

The principles are:

1) To prioritize the setting you are to serve in the world. Do this through reflection. Release the outcome and expectations of others who have a predetermined way of what you are to do and how you are to do it.

2) Allow spirituality to become known. The world is ready for this reflection and it will greatly accelerate the understanding of what is available.

3) Rededicate your life to the mission and then become one pointed in all that you do.

4) There is need to rest and renew the self at deep levels in order to work more from the spiritual perspective rather than the personality.

5) Refrain from speaking unkindly to those who are slower to believe in themselves and be patient and trust that all will happen as planned and within the destiny of one's life purpose. There have been some trappings that have gotten you off center. Reflect on the past to see more clearly and wait for guidelines for future action within and without.

6) Reshape consciousness of the world, to take this challenge seriously and find the answers to the multiplicity of time and space including multidimensional living.

7) Remember to care for the self in all ways to have the energy to do the work easily for that is how you will know that you are on track.

I go now.

Lovingly, Mary

Recorded by Mary Jo Bulbrook (3/13/94, Christchurch, NZ)

Stay on the Path
Dear one,

Be not mistaken, time is running out in which to approach the Divine perspective. Do not falter from the path save yourself without regard to explore inner and outer dimensions. There is richness that awaits all those who follow the path and choose to not waver from its' Divine perspective.

Coming to you and exploring all of the dimensions available to search your internal clock enriches me. Find you center more readily and we will be able to come to you more readily. The things that are bugging you a re not of your making but rather come of outer awareness impinging on your growth. Stay on the Path.

Lovingly, Mary
Recorded by Mary Jo Bulbrook (6/94)

The Mystical Power of Prayer

I wanted to include a translation from Aramaic to English of the "Our Father" that was sent to me via e-mail in October 1999, and relate the message of the prayer to the philosophy of the Energetic Healing Program. Dan, the editor, and I decided against it, since we did not have the original source of the prayer.

A few weeks later I found a copy of a book titled, *Prayers of the Cosmos: Meditations on the Aramaic Words of Jesus* (by Neil Douglas-Klotz) mysteriously lying on the top of my bed. I picked it up and realized the book was a birthday present to me by the coordinator of the Energetic Healing program last year. As I write this, I finally opened to the power of what was being given to me.

The process I am describing is how God works as one's life is turned over to God. Many things take place that are interrelated and part of a larger plan for you. You have choices to make. When those choices are in alignment with God, the flow, power, and synchronicity and peace are tremendous. My goal in sharing this piece is to pass on the mystical power of prayer that is available to all of us as we begin to pray with reverence.

Although I am focusing on the words of Jesus, which are part of my spiritual tradition, there are similar prayers and teachings in other traditions. One only needs to search their heritage to find "power prayers" to connect with and use. Finding meaning and value in life is critical to all healing. The task of a healer is to create a framework to help a person find their spiritual Light.

As one says the prayer, the intention is to experience the vibrations, or to have what Klotz says are body prayers encouraging a person, "To participate in the sound and feeling of the words as well as their intellectual or metaphorical meaning." (p. 4) In other words, to experience the mystical or universal level of interpretation, Klotz says, "I feel that the need of the earth is so great that we must do everything helpful to reestablish harmony with all creation." (p. 4)

Many of you are familiar with the King James Version (Matthew 6:9-13) of the Lord's Prayer. I will also share one version of the New Translation from the Aramaic from Neil Douglas-Klotz and relate the original meaning of the words of Jesus to the philosophy behind the Energetic Healing Program.

The Lord's Prayer
(Matthew 6: 9-13, King James Version)
Our Father which art in heaven
Hallowed be thy name.
Thy kingdom come.
Thy will be done on earth, as it is in heaven.
Give us this day our daily bread.
And forgive us our debts, as we forgive our debtors.
And lead us not into temptation, but deliver us from evil.
For thine is the kingdom, and the power, and the glory, forever.
Amen.

One Aramaic Version from Neil Douglas Klotz (p.41, 1990)
O Birther! Father-Mother of the Cosmos,
Focus your Light within us — make it useful:
Create your reign of unity now —
Your one desire then acts with ours,
As in all Light, so in all forms.
Grant what we need each day in bread and insight.
Loose the cords of mistakes binding us,
As we release the strands we hold of others' guilt.
Don't let surface things delude us,
But free us from what holds us back.
From you is born all ruling will,
The power and the life to do,
The song that beautifies all,
From age to age it renews.
Truly — power to these statements —
may they be the ground from which all my actions grow.
Amen.

I believe that the holiness of the experience is directly proportion-
ate to the spiritual awareness that a individual gives to the act of
praying. There is the rote recitation of prayers and there is the full
energy experience of it. I noticed the difference in this process as I
witnessed the various priests giving the sign of the cross after a
Catholic mass. The priests that engage the energy of the signing with
an energetic expression of faith actually send healing energies to
those who are ready to receive. If one stays in an open state, the
blessing is fully integrated. If not, the blessing is like water off of a

ducks back, it hits the surface of our energy and then is washed off. My whole process when I am in a religious ceremony now is to attune to the energy dynamics. I have experienced varied things.

The philosophy of the Energetic Healing Program encompasses the Father-Mother, male-female energies. The command to focus your light within and make it useful is a clear mandate to work on spiritual dimensions. The act of, "loosing the cords of mistakes that bind us and releasing others' guilt" is the major focus of the EH "Healing Wounds" class. When we don't forgive, we hold others at a lower spiritual plane and this in turn affects our light and love. "Be free from what holds us back," relates to changing the beliefs that do not serve your soul's purpose.

My experience of being drawn to report this prayer is yet one example of how the spiritual flow had played out in my life in this instance regarding my chosen task to serve the healing community by passing on the stories of light and love, and the development of oneness with Spirit. A solid prayer life that is done with intention sets the tone for the healing process. As a healer operates from this process by attuning to the Divine, there is a very deep spiritual awakening that is possible flooding one's being with light and love, the two ingredients of healing.

Mary Jo Bulbrook
Carrboro, North Carolina

LUX AETERNA
(Eternal Light)

Long after sun disappears
eternal lamp stays lit.
Foundation of life
it shines invisible:
We all walk in its protection,
dream in it, cast no shadow;
live out our entire lives,
perhaps unaware,
perhaps rejoicing that it's there.

Roger Weinstein
Atlanta, GA

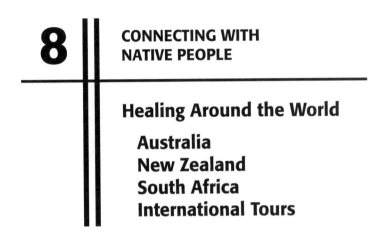

8 | **CONNECTING WITH NATIVE PEOPLE**

Healing Around the World
Australia
New Zealand
South Africa
International Tours

Introduction: A Prophesy Comes True

In 1976 I attended a meeting with a group of colleagues associated with Virginia Satir, internationally renowned family therapist. A social worker from Australia told the group about her work with the Aborigines. A strange feeling came over me as I listened to her. I felt as if I were in a time warp and not fully present. I sensed that I would some day be working with the Aborigines! Since I had never heard about Aborigines before, I wondered what this feeling may mean. I did not say anything to my friends at the time. I registered the feeling in my "energy system," a concept that I did not use at that point in my career.

Years later I entered the holistic health field and studied new versions of old traditions in energy-based healing. I first studied Therapeutic Touch with Dolores Krieger in 1976, then Touch for Health in 1978. I developed Healing From Within and Without in 1986 (my own Holistic Nursing Theory). I studied Healing Touch in 1990 plus a few other modalities thrown in between.

In 1990 I accepted a Visiting Professor position at Edith Cowan University in Perth, Western Australia to teach nursing research. I "knew" that I was to go there, but I heard a "voice" that instructs me to accept only a one year position rather than the three year position I was offered. As I prepare to go with hesitancy, I sense things are going to happen to change the course of my life.

I offered an introduction to Healing Touch to the University and nursing community that was received with cautious eyes. My work is filmed by the university media department under the able direction of David Crewes. After I left the Memorial University if Newfoundland in 1987, I wished I could work where they have a good media department to produce educational media to teach the kind of things I am interested in. To my luck, but not surprise, as I am now used to Spirit working in my life, I landed at a university that has one of the best media departments in Australia. This event set the stage for access to develop resources using media to capture the magic of energy-based modalities in a seven-set video series called, "Healing From Within and Without" (which became the basis for my Energetic Healing program). In Australia I also had the opportunity to film my work which combined energy-based therapies with Virginia Satir's family therapy in a film series called, "Helping Individuals and Families Change."

Throughout the time I was in Western Australia for that one-year position teaching nursing research, I searched throughout the university community for a link to the "vague feeling" I had in 1976 about working with Aborigines. When nothing turned up I began to wonder about that premonition. I just kept trusting that if something were to come of the my intuition I would know when it came true.

I completed my year and returned to the USA wondering if anything would happen. I knew I would to return to Australia. The one year at the University in Australia enabled me to learn about international travel and develop connections in international health care. Up to that point I was minimally knowledgeable, but I was familiar with the Canadian system having spent six years as professor responsible for the graduate nursing program at the Memorial University of Newfoundland.

By 1992, I was an instructor in Healing Touch and answered a call to help Janet Mentgen "do her work" of spreading HT worldwide. I received this message during the first HT class that I took in Durham, NC. To this day, I honor that spiritual directive.

Even though I was not fully aware of it then, my destiny was being shaped by spiritual links. In retrospect, I am able to see the pieces fit together. My name is given to the organizing committee in New Zealand for a international conference that had a mission to connect people worldwide in healing with an objective of honoring the indigenous people and their teaching. Several obstacles presented themselves to me to attend that conference, but I have an "energy push" to overcome them. Learning to trust guidance and stay on target is a constant calling and challenge.

At that international gathering, I met Bob Randall, a native Australian Aborigine, and Rose Pere, a Maori Tohuna (spiritual teacher) of New Zealand. The three of us vowed to stay connected and share our common paths of healing and teaching healing through the wisdom of our cultural background. All three of us are spiritually focused in everything we do. Bob, Rose, and I soon became "family" and remain close to this day.

These experiences continually show the evolution of the healer. There is no set path that you control. You only walk as far as you can see, and once you reach a horizon, a new one opens to show the next step of the way. Healing Touch becomes the connecting link for Bob, Rose and I to organize our lives around. However the real connection is through Spirit—answering the call to heal and to teach the ancient wisdom.

Mary Jo Bulbrook
Carrboro, North Carolina

FULFILLING DESTINY IN AUSTRALIA

Aborigine Connections: Bob Randall

I identified in the preceding story, "A Prophesy Come True," that meeting Bob Randall, an Aborigine from Central Australia, was part of my destiny predicted in 1976, when I had a "feeling" I was going to do something with the Aborigines. Bob and I met in Christchurch, New Zealand and we "danced" around each other energetically many times before finally connecting. We were thrown together socially on several occasions. Bob would come to the gathering with his guitar and be the center of attention. He was soft-spoken, yet he commanded a great presence.

I would describe Bob as having soft, gentle, humble, feminine energy and a quick sense of humor demonstrated by his ability to laugh at himself. I would find myself standing next to Bob in the food lines and feeling his "presence." I soon realized that he was all too familiar to me. His energy seemed to match mine—we were as "one," a very comfortable unit. It all seemed very strange to me to experience this black man from so far away. I am sure he felt the same!

One night while we were holding hands in a circle of people at a Marae, the meeting place of the Maori, I had a vision of walking the land, long ago with Bob as my partner. It was an odd feeling, yet I felt so natural and at home too. I could feel the land under my feet, see the scenery, and feel the presence of his hand in mine. From that day forward I knew Bob was tied into the "vague feeling" I had years ago of what I was destined to experience.

Bob came to the workshop I gave in Christchurch and said, "You are doing what our people did long ago. I want you to come and help me with my people." From that day forward I made a commitment to work with Bob and help his people.

The exact form this connection would take was not yet clear, so we just walked our path and went as far as our feet and vision would take us. I told Bob that I knew a lot of my people who would also like to connect with his people. This was the beginning of my intent to bring tours to Australia and connect with the Aborigines.

When I returned to the states after meeting Bob, three people at separate times asked me if I had read, *Mutant Message Down Under*. I had not read it but realized with so many people asking me, I needed to read it! So I went out and bought M. Morgan's book and felt as if I was reading about something very familiar. I came across the section that said two people had been together before and made a decision to come back together as they had something to do together. Only they agreed that they would only meet after fifty years had passed. I had just turned fifty when I met Bob so I knew that book was also talking about me!

In those early days, I did not know who Bob really was, although I "knew" him on a deeper level. Over the years I learned of his gifts as a storyteller, singer and songwriter, digideridoo player, teacher, healer and keeper of the Aborigine sacred traditions.

In 1999, Bob received the distinguished award of "Aborigine Man of the Year." He was committed to speak his truth and share the knowledge of land and culture. He was one of the "lost generation" of Aborigines removed from his family when he was quite young and placed in an orphanage to be raised in the "white ways." He never saw his mother again. He is registered as one as traditional owners of Uluru, the sacred Aboriginal name for Ayers Rock. Bob is of the Pitjantjatjara tribe.

In the 70's NBC did a story of Bob's life. In 1998 while touring once again in Central Australia, we got in on the tail end of a new film updating his life by the same company that aired his story all across Australia. You can see and recognize Donna Duff at least three times in the film!

There are times when I have spontaneously turned on the TV in U.S. and saw Bob's smiling face looking at me. He is one of the key people contacted to relate the Aborigine stories. Currently he is completing a book on his life that will be published in 2000.

So that is who Bob Randall is, how we met, and how we came together!

Mary Jo Bulbrook
Carrboro, North Carolina

The Aborigine Way

When I was a child, I lived in a home without walls. This was my *ngura*, my country. The stars were the ceiling of my house and the earth was the floor. The horizon was just the entrance to another room. Nothing separated me from the wind, the heat and the cold, or the sounds of the birds and insects that lived in my country. For seven precious years I lived like this, and through the stories told to me as we walked through country, or sat around the fire at night, this landscape and everything in it were my intimate family, my *waltja*, or kinship system.

With open space living like this, there is a bigness. A hugeness. And it is such a good feeling because you feel part of everything you see. From that very early time as a child, this bigness was part of me, and everything out there that I could see, smell, hear, and feel was all part of me. I was all of everything that was around me. The land I lived on, sat on, ran on, was there because my flesh was touching it, and I could reach out to any plant at any time or pick a grass or a flower or a stone. It was a feeling of belonging that was so strong. It was a fantastic feeling of being in control of the universe in a way that you felt part of that universe. It wasn't something separate from you because it was part of your moment by moment living.

To the Aborigines, time is not linear. We practise *kanyini* in the four dimensions of reality—mind, body, spirit, and land so as to maintain holistic well-being, not just for ourselves, but for everything around us. When we misuse any of these dimensions, we lose our well-being, in ourselves, our community, and our environment. Kanyini is the principle of connectedness through caring and responsibility that underpins Aboriginal life. Kanyini links four main areas of responsibility—*tjukurrpa* (philosophy, law and religion), *ngura* (country), *walytja* (kinship and family) and *kurunpa* (spirit, soul and psyche).

Tjukurrpa is creation, the one time in the beginning when all things were created, and which we need to keep alive in the present. Not only the land forms and the original plants, insects, reptiles and birds, but the social laws, the lore, which we have to live by. All this comes from tjukurrpa. This is the bigger consciousness of something that was, and is, the way to live in harmony with all things. Living this is a matter of how we do things in the present. So when we think about time, it is only the now, the present that is important. Each and every moment of nowness is where we live out the truth of the connectedness of kanyini.

There is us, as people, but this was never a restricting thing because "people" is all of us. Right throughout my life, old men would point to a forest of trees or a grove of trees or just one tree and refer to it as people. "See that mob over there," could be referring to kangaroos, trees, hills or humans. Any of us could be "that mob" or us mob could include the totality of that. Throughout my life I discovered, from other Aboriginal groups with whom I have lived, that having the idea of connecting with all things was quite common throughout the different Aboriginal nations.

There is such a gulf between the traditional Aboriginal way of understanding reality and the way white society seems to. For us, everything is intimately interconnected. But white people separate things out, even the relationship between their minds and their bodies, but especially between themselves and other people and nature. For example, they have one sort of doctor who fixes the body, and another sort of doctor who fixes the mind, and yet another sort of person who is responsible for spirit. And none of these sorts of people have anything to do with responsibility for country. This in turn is split up between people who use the land, like farmers, pastoralists and miners, or people who look after nature like environmentalists and national park and wildlife rangers. This seems really crazy to our way of thinking and experiencing reality.

Through opening up our inner eye and through deep, quiet listening and awareness, we can learn to communicate with the land as our mother, with the trees and the elements, and with all the other creatures who are our "family." From this experience of profound inter-being, we are able to understand how to recover the energy of kanyini and use this to transform our lives, and the lives of those around us.

Our line of Aboriginal healers are known as *nungaries*. They are trained from an early age, when we recognise the ability of a healer in a child and nurture that child and train him to use it for good and not the other way, for sorcery. In Central Australia today, traditional healers, nungaries, work side by side with modern western doctors. They are particularly effective in dealing with sickness of spirit which is behind a seemingly only physical illness. For example, there was a little boy who was brought to the hospital in a state of listlessness and depression. They could not see anything physically wrong with him so they called the nungarie. Immediately he recognised that the boy's spirit was not there. He questioned the parents and discovered the child had undergone a severe fright during a game. So the white doctor and the nungarie returned to the place where this had happened, and the nungarie found the spirit and took it back to the hospital where he returned the spirit to the child. The boy then recovered quite quickly.

Healing is done in a moment, it does not take a lot of time. In some cases all it takes is a smile or gentle word. The healing way is done by your inner self, by your mind, and by your touch. These are the three elements—inner self, mind, and touch—and all are controlled by thought. Think well about each other. Here is an exercise to try. I want you to think about the words you would have liked most to hear, which would have made you feel good most of the time. I want you to whisper to the person on either side of you those words. Whisper those words you would have wanted someone to say to you most of the time about yourself, coming from the concept that you are a beautiful being, that you always have been and you always will be. I'll give you a few minutes to do that.

Did everyone speak to someone in a whisper? Healing is as gentle as that. It starts with someone saying something nice. And the sickness will start the other way, saying something that is not nice. Saying it, publicizing it, implementing it in the publicity of policy and it can effect and influence the whole of society. There is a way to change that by starting with ourselves. I've got to think of myself as having value—value enough to care.

All things are also part of your families. The tree is no different from you. If you cut me and I cut you, we both bleed. If we cut the tree, it also bleeds. If you tune into the interconnectedness of nature through the dimension of spirit, you can feel this. That closeness is family (waltja), it is relationship (kanyini). So our learning was that a person was only allowed to take so much of a tree that is needed to break the wind at night and nothing more. When my family used to camp in the desert amongst the sand hills—you wouldn't cut down the whole tree because you have to consider its rights as well.

Even the plants for food we treat the same way. There is a very popular honey we get out of the ground taken from the honey ants (tjala). The honey ant has his home there. You can take a lot but you don't take all of it. You always leave some there. And especially you leave the workers, which is good economic planning, isn't it? The same way with the plants that are taken for tuba, roots and vegetables. You just dig another hole on the side and put the plant in again. They are always there. You never take the whole.

As teenagers we made some mistakes like all children will. I would like to share these mistakes with you as a warning to all young people. In Arnhem Land, during the turtle mating season, the turtle is not allowed to be taken as food. You have to leave it alone regardless of how hungry you may be. This is the law. One day we went looking for something to eat and did not find anything. We were coming back with our spears over our shoulders and someone said, "Hey look at that water splashing out there." The waves were coming in and there is a lot of noise going on, a lot of action. We looked and saw that the turtles were mating. The friends I was with said, "Well what do you reckon?" We restrained ourselves at first because we knew that you cannot take the turtle at mating time, but we had nothing to eat. A second day went and now we were really hungry. The oldest of my friends said, "Let's take our chances with it. The elders are ten miles away near the Mission, so no one will know." So we sneaked up close and because they were mating, they took no notice of us. We got a big one, brought it in, cooked it, ate it, and buried everything. We congratulated ourselves, "Oh, that was really good." We rested awhile and headed back home.

As we approached home, what was waiting for us but three of the elders, standing and staring from the cliff top. The way they were looking at us, we knew we were in trouble. One said to us, "Did any of you boys do anything wrong?" We said, "No." We wondered how he knew! He asked, "What did you boys do that for, what have you done?" And we said again, "Did what? Did what, Uncle?" He said, "You all killed that turtle and you shouldn't have." "Don't you know the birds were watching? Those birds told us."

We were punished with the profound sense of guilt that is often the beginning of illness, because it affects the spirit. We knew it was wrong, yet still we did it. So our spirit was weak with the sadness of breaking the kanyini which linked us to the turtle and our tjukurrpa laws. Our traditional belief is that if you break the law, it can cause illness this way.

It is the same if other laws are broken, like trespassing in a woman's ceremony. Women have their ceremony each year in the places they pick where no men are allowed. Now if any men intrude on this area, we're in trouble. We have broken the law. In the same way, the men's ceremony on ceremonial grounds becomes sacred on the completion of the ceremony for quite some time because the land holds the memory of this. You must leave it alone when its ongoing and you can't even go near it when it's finished. If you violate that law there is big trouble.

Our law is established in a kinship, family way. Every single person within a tribe is family and related through that kinship system. It's like, say, all of us here today would be one tribe. Under the holistic healing, we are one tribe, we are one family and we are all related caring for and about each other, each with the good in mind and heart for the family. And so should not hurt each other.

Bob Randal
Central Australia

Walking the Land for Direction

Bob and I had many conversations about what we were being guided to do together. He always would tell me, "I need to walk the land and get guidance." It was from this that I learned the importance of the process of walking the land that is key to all indigenous people.

Bob had picked out a spot that was about 15 minutes outside of Alice Springs in Central Australia for our work. The property belonged to his daughter's husband's "mob" as the tribes are affectionately called! One day I was there with Bob, he was very excited about showing me the site he picked out for our work together.

He and I were alone walking the land just like in the old days. Bob pointed in one direction and said, "Look at how beautiful this is." He turned to the other side and said, "I must be able to see these trees, no matter what I do." Then he walked over to a central place and said, "Here is one spot." We were there a while, feeling the energy. He then walked forward to another spot with the intention for me to follow him. As I walked away, I heard a voice that said this is the gathering place. I yelled to Bob that I heard a voice saying this was to be the gathering place. His reply was, "Don't make up your mind yet, there is more that I want to show you!"

He took me to a magnificent gum tree. There were not many trees around. I looked around and did not see anything. As I leaned up against the tree to feel it's energy and look at the peak in front of me, I saw someone caring for someone on a table, high up on a steep, stone hill. As I squinted my eyes and looked up, I wondered what it meant and how they got up there? With that, the vision came down before my eyes and landed right next to me. I shouted with excitement, "Bob, this is where we are to do the nurturing, the caring for people." Bob replied, "Don't make up your mind yet, I have another place to show you."

We walked to another gum tree. I once again leaned against the tree and felt again the energy flow from the tree up into my body. As I looked up I saw a group of Aborigine men. I wondered what they were doing up there and what that meant. I realized that Aborigine men and woman do things separately. The other place was the woman's business, for nurturing and caring. This place was for men's business, for ceremony, as that is the role of Aborigine men. Again I shouted to Bob. After showing me each place, he would go off by himself and sit in the bush to absorb the energies.

As we walked toward the trees I heard a voice from the tree that said the ancestors and spirits were among the trees and watching what we were doing. They would oversee the project regarding our joint venture. That is the reason Bob kept insisting that we keep the view of the trees in sight at all times.

Bob took a stick and drew in the land what we walked. It was a triangle of 1. Gathering Place, 2. Nurturing Place for Healing (women), and 3. Ceremony for Planning (men). All three parts were connected together. Hence was born, following ancient tradition, the form for our healing/teaching center of the Aborigine/Healing Touch Partnership.

Mary Jo Bulbrook
Carrboro, North Carolina

Healing Journeys: We Are All One

As a coastal dweller I had always wondered what it would be like to go to the Red Center (Uluru – Ayers Rock). I decided to join HT Partnerships to connect with the land, meet Bob Randall and his family, and learn more about Aborigine healing traditions, as well as sharing our healing work with them.

As we were flying in to Alice I had this very curious feeling like I was coming home. Bob met us at the airport and after taking our things to the resort, he took us out to walk the land. On the walk we saw the Amphitheater, which is a rocky ridge shaped like a beautiful rainbow that sheltered the land from the south and west. We walked on, along the dry riverbed to the next rock outcrop of pink quartz. As we approached this rock I felt very strange: anxious, teary, and my thyroid was pounding. I said this to Bob and he explained that this was the Heart Stone where you come to contemplate the past and say good-bye to lost family and friends. To me this was a profound demonstration of connecting with the land, as I had come to HT through the death of my father and my own need to heal around the consequences of his death. In that moment I felt relieved, blessed, and grateful to my father for having prompted this journey.

Over the next few days, as the journey unfolded and our sacred purpose for coming together revealed itself, Mary Jo, Donna, Bob, and I connected on a level that is only possible through mutual sharing of experiences that are both simple, profound, and enlightening. We traveled to sacred sights, performed traditional rituals to heal the relationships between the land, the animals that inhabit it, and the humans, one to another. We connected to heal, and we were healed. It was a wonderful blessing to be part of Aborigine family, the land, and the journey.

I came to understand, once and for all, that as we heal ourselves, we contribute to the greater whole and help heal the entire planet. This brings true meaning to the passing of a loved one. Thanks Dad. Love, Sue.

Sue Pattinson
Wauchope, New South Wales, Australia

Healing Hands Aborigine Drawing

While in Central Australia in 1995, I had commissioned an Aborigine to design a picture for me to use in my work. Bob and I met with an Aborigine artist and described our work together. We hoped that he would create a drawing that captured the vision of our work. The time came and went, and there was no Aborigine design. At first I was irritated and upset, but soon settled into an acceptance and said,

"I wonder why this is not working? There must be something else in store for us!"

I was scheduled to teach HT Level I and IIA in Denmark, Western Australia in February 1996. At the last minute the level IIA did not make. The coordinators said to me, "I wonder what is in store for us with having an extra two days." During the time in Denmark some magical things happened to me. While I was teaching one of the participants told me about this Aborigine healer who had worked on her partner doing readings by playing the didjeridoo over the body. The Didjeridoo is an instrument from the top end of Australia and is really a man's instrument. Women are not suppose to play them, but in this case playing them for healing was OK.

I was given the opportunity to go see this woman healer on my two free days. We made an appointment to go to her place where she saw clients and had a craft shop with Aborigine paintings and other things. When we arrived I was struck with the power of the place. I took a photograph of a magnificent tree in her yard. When it was developed there was an spirit visible in the leaf area of the picture. Then I knew why I was so drawn to the place!

As I walked into the shop, Maxine looked at me straight into the eyes and called me "sister." She made such intense contact with my soul that I could not look away. We shared many stories and were invited into her home for a cup of tea with her family. It was like being at home not half way around the world in an Aborigine's home!

Maxine did a personal reading for me. After the reading I was telling her about my desire to have an Aborigine artist draw something to show the connection between Healing Touch Partnerships and the Aborigines in our work together. I shared my disappointment that the original artist did not follow through on his commitment.

As I spoke, Maxine received images and said that she would be happy to do it for me! We talked further as I described my work and I left with her promise to create a painting that I could use in my work. Maxine is an artist renowned throughout Australia. Her works are in shops everywhere. Of course she was the one to do the painting and was waiting for me to find her. Maxine is not only a healer but an artist and a nurse! Needless to say, it was clear that we were destined to work together.

I was amazed when Maxine sent me the painting and wrote up the description of what it meant. Aborigines use the same language as we do! Her description follows:

The two figures in the Center of the picture represent Spirit Woman dancing. They are without rivalry and pride or negative sentiment in any way, so in fact they are naked. Naked of all self— only the deep love and oneness with all women and purity that continually motivated them to be human channels of Healing, Peace, and Light. Light because they have emptied themselves of All darkness. In their coming together they give the golden light of All totalness—the Gold of the morning then the Gold of the evening, and in the night, Complete Rest.

The Water Holes of Life: We are reminded by the symbols that WE are nurtured, Physically, Mentally, Emotionally and Spiritually at all times and continually remind ourselves of this our own self-esteem.

Web of Life: Holding the Weaker one giving support and guidance until the Weaker becomes strong. She in turn becomes strong. To the help another one and so on—until our lands, people, minds, and nations are healed.

Dots tell of Equality: We are equal to everything, the Wind, the Sun, the Moon, and the Trees because were are a part of everything we see. This is particularly true for healers whose awareness and recognition of elements of deeper principles unable them to also be elements, channels, and givers of healing love.

The overall painting is in the symbol of a larger Circle. The symbol as we give, we receive and always the cycle continues—the more we give, we receive—the need to be aware of the sacredness of our being here now at this time . . . to be apart of this world's change for the better.

With My Blessings,
Maxine Fumagalli, Aborigine Healer
Denmark, Western Australia (7/17/96)

The painting was presented to me within six months and was packed for the long journey back to America where the original sits in my office. I see it every day I am home.

Mary Jo Bulbrook
Carrboro, North Carolina

Aborigine Messages

Throughout my experiences in Australia there were many magical things that happened to me. In order to record them, I created cards called Aborigine Messages, that represent Aborigines sacred teachings or messages I received as I walked the land. Some are recorded below for you to meditate on. The most important one relates the signing of the agreement between the Aborigines and me for the Healing Touch Partnership Property site. That saying is: Respect the land, respect the people, respect the practices at all times.

Honor the mysteries. Honor the elders. Honor the healers.

Service multiplies one's powers.

The tribe has the responsibility to maintain the songs, stories, dance and the role of totems.

Stand in the footprints of the person in front of you to experience them.

Live from the inner still place. What is inside is all that is needed.

Record the stories. Share them, to pass on our truths, so many will understand.

Call people in by your songs and lighten their hearts.

Songlines are based on teachings of ancient spirits. Pick up their energy from the land. Families are expected to pass on knowledge and culture through ritual and ceremony. The best foods are what are in season and cared for in ceremony.

We are only limited by our ability to notice.

Take information into the ear and hear it in your heart.

Losing the land, we lose part of ourselves as we are of the land.

To visit spiritual sites, we must prepare ourselves.

Listen to those who have gone before you.

Mary Jo Bulbrook
Carrboro, North Carolina

JOURNEY TO NEW ZEALAND

First Visit to New Zealand

I had been invited to teach HT in New Zealand by one of the presenters I met at the American Holistic Nurses' Association meeting in 1994. Sonja was a nurse from Auckland. We had talked about my visiting her country to teach HT. She had come to our country to recruit someone to offer some additional healing modalities. I agreed to go and set out for my first visit.

When I arrived, my host took me to one of her favorite places to meditate. We both went our separate ways to meditate alone. I had one of the most significant visions of my life. I saw a group of light beings surrounding some vehicle. They were encased in shimmering light that was pulsating. They told me what I was about to do in NZ was very important and they would be watching me! When Sonja returned I told her about what I saw. She looked at me and with polite attention directed me back to the car. I could tell that she was wondering about me!

I remember the first time I saw light beings was while I was learning to teach IIIA with Janet Mentgen. Since I was not in charge of the classroom, my awareness was on watching the energy dynamics in the room without having to focus on any particular thing. Behind the group I saw a picture of light beings in spirit form like the cover of Barbara Brennan's *Hands of Light*! I remember the first time I saw Barbara's book, my first words were, "I am glad that she can do that. There is no way I could ever do that." Now here it was several years later and I was indeed seeing light beings.

We went to another place that was a tourist information center. It overlooked a beautiful garden area and port. Once again she went in one direction and I in the other. This time an Egyptian woman appeared to me laid out on a couch! I laughed at myself and said. "An Egyptian woman on a couch?" When I said this, she turned to me in a disgusted voice and said, "I watch over the land. I need to tell you to tell the people they must start honoring the land." She then turned away from me.

Sonja returned and I told her again what I saw. She looked at me with even greater disbelief and I thought to myself that I had better shut up or I would be in deep trouble! We went to a beach and were lying on the sand. It was a very significant beach, one that there are many postcards about! There was a shaft of land jutting out of the water. As I causally looked up at this, I saw an Indian standing on the top. In disbelief, I squinted my eyes and thought to myself, an Indian? He looked down at me and said that his role was to watch those that came into the land and warn others if there was danger!

Yes, I did it again, I told Sonja what I saw. This was the final blow as the look on her face said that I went too far. I laughed, as there was nothing else that I could do! We went off to her home and I knew I had some new things in store for me in New Zealand!

It was this same trip that I met Rose Pere and Bob Randall in Christchurch, NZ. We were speakers at an international conference. Meeting Rose and Bob is described elsewhere in this book, but what I want to tell you about in this story is that I told Rose about my visions starting with the Egyptian woman. She said indeed the Maori people are directly connected to Egypt. It is no accident that I saw her and it was not unusual! I gave a sigh of relief to find out that I was not crazy or maybe we both were. Anyway, she also said that the connections with Indians is there as well. Her people are direct links to all the indigenous people of the world. Throughout the years I have traveled many times to NZ and met with Rose, and her family.

The native people have taken me into realms I never would attempt to go, much less imagine I would ever experience. Following my path as a healer and answering my call has opened many new doors for me. New paths will open for you too as you connect with your spiritual guidance and destiny as a soul to fulfill your life's purpose.

I have chosen to be frank about what happened to me because I feel the need to support budding healers whom are just starting on this path. Your life will change as mine changed. *It will change in the proportion to the risks you take.* And yes, you will lose some people along the way that will not be able to handle your changes! Trust me though, it has been worth it!

Mary Jo Bulbrook
Carrboro, North Carolina

Maori Connection: Rose Pere

My first connection with Rose in New Zealand is an interesting story. She was staying with a friend of the woman I was staying with, Mavis Jean, who I met in the USA during my HT Level IV training. Mavis Jean was my partner for the instructor's course. That night on our way to a pot luck dinner we stopped to pick up something to bring. I was in the back seat and Rose was in the front seat. A woman appeared to me and indicated she wanted to get a message to Rose. I was very surprised and more cautious how I would introduce this "far out vision" to someone I did not know. Rose is a distinguish elder in the Maori culture and I felt as if I was in the presence of "royalty." Nonetheless, I gathered my courage and told her what I experienced. She was not surprised and began to ask me a series of questions about the vision.

As Rose asked a question, I would get the information. Rose is also very super sensitive and perceptive. One of her roles in her culture is to link with the spirits of her people and serve as a spiritual healer. The woman that appeared to me had lost her child and was in anguish. After I made the identification of the vision that she could link with, Rose did her "thing" and launched into her Maori tradition of healing. As I sat back and listened to Rose, I wondered where all of this would take me.

This was the beginning of many spiritual connections with Rose that would span many years. In 1997, Rose would travel with me, Bob, and 28 other healers teaching Healing Touch and indigenous healing throughout the USA and Canada. We would also speak at the American Holistic Nurses' Association, the International Society for the Study of Subtle Energy and Energy Medicine in Boulder, CO, and the International Congress of Nurses in Vancouver, BC. Wherever we traveled, our classes and energy blended native teaching and ancient wisdom with Healing Touch.

Mary Jo Bulbrook
Carrboro, North Carolina

Healing from the Heart with Love: A Maori Perspective

A A A A A A A A A I I I I I I I I I I O O O O O O O O O O O

A (ah)   The Divine Mother on my left.
I (ee)   The Divine Child, the Inner Being in the centre of me.
O (or)   The Divine Father on my right.

I send you my love,
as I feel your sacred reflection
in the mirror of my heart.

The Mirror of My heart

Left	Centre	Right
A	I	O
Divine Mother	Divine Child	Divine Father
	Sacred River	
	Sacred Seed	

From The Central Sun,
The Divine Spark
Ira Tangata (Human Being)

I   Child (from the)
Ra   Central Sun, Divine Spark
Ta   Blue print, D.N.A.; from the Godhead
nga   Breath from the Godhead
ta   Hologram of the Godhead

The energy of New Zealand is "AROHA," the presence and the breath of the Godhead, unconditional love. May our constant companion during this gathering be AROHA. Our mountains, our rivers, our lakes, our glaciers, our hot pools, our forest lands, everything that uplifts the oneness of all things also extend their greetings of AROHA to everyone who is present.

A common form of greeting in New Zealand is "KIA ORA" in its ordinary meaning, and yet the depth of sacred meaning is awesome, in that it also conveys the following energy, and vibrations:

            K   IAO   RA

K   subtle vibration
I   the Divine Child
A   the Divine Mother
O   the Divine Father (from)
RA the Central Sun, the Divine Spark

Two thirds of our communication in Maori is completely abstract, to the point that people who learn our language fluently, may only learn about ordinary meaning, but not sacred meaning. Our ancient teachings are transmitted by the *Tohuna* (keepers of the secrets who know when and how to sow the seeds). These types of people are born into families who have the "key" to the higher schools of learning on the upper twelve planes.

Prior to January 14th, 1990, when the alignment of Turuki (the North Star), and Rehua (the smallest star in the Southern Cross) took place, I would not have been able to share much of what I have shared with you today. The Tohuna have great discipline, and although there were many challenges to give away the sacred teachings before the appropriate time, our people managed to keep everything intact until the given time. What we basically shared with the Europeans prior to 1990, were divinations including mythology that was akin to what the Europeans spoke about in terms of themselves. In this way, the Europeans could not interfere with our "ancient path" and disrupt the continuity of sacred transmission.

When the Europeans came to New Zealand they spoke about the Father and the Son in their religious teachings, so the Maori told them about "IO," and hid the vibration of "A," the Mother. From the ancient Maori to the present time we realize the importance of linking in to the oneness of all things. In fact when we are in perfect harmony, we can tune in with, and indeed become, the stars, the trees, the coral reefs, the dolphins, the sun, the moon, and anything we need to become, in order to help with the process of healing; whether it be with people, with other living things, with Earth Mother, or with other planets and galaxies.

Spiritual healing always precedes physical healing, healing which may include massaging, herbal medicines, sound and vibration, water, kumara (sweet potato), stone, anything that may reveal itself as the appropriate agent for "cleansing." What some cultures may refer to as disease or illness is referred to as "cleansing" in the Maori makeup, in that the person or persons involved have to find out what has happened on a spiritual level to invoke the type of "cleansing" that is experienced. Some people can experience the same type of cleansing several times over because they have not truly understood how they have gone against the natural belief system they were born with to clear themselves on the spiritual planes.

We also recognize and accept other forms of healing that may be brought into our space from another culture. To us the most important part of healing is to feel and have faith in the power of unconditional love that comes from the Godhead. Right now I am traversing on spiritual planes above the "eighth" and am aware that my physical body needs help to keep up with the frequency changes. I would appreciate the healing power of those present to help me overcome some "cleansing," in my legs particularly.

The potential of healing is in every person. The assumption is that every person is born with great wisdom and great power, because s/he is the essence of the Godhead, AIO. European Christian missionaries came to the Maori in New Zealand quite convinced they had to save the Maori from damnation. This attitude still exists in some circles.

We also have other people, including spiritual healers, trying to teach us how to adjust to the so called "New Age" and how we need to cleanse our sacred places! It has not yet entered their heads that we, the Maori, have been the Keepers of the "South Pacific Rim of Fire" for thousands of years as decreed by our ancient forebears. We have never let the fires die out by "hordes of darkness" either, as suggested by some so called "gurus." In fact, the fires are burning brighter than ever, in that some of us have always chosen to be Warriors For Peace, even against great odds. We refer to gatherings that took place over five billion years ago because we know that the spirits we have are very ancient. Sometimes we refer to other cultures as our "senior brothers and sisters" to be polite, but on a spiritual level, no one is more senior or junior.

Another wonderful thing is that people basically heal themselves once they put their minds to it, although other people can come in alongside to help them remember how to call on their own energy and other energy flows that can help. Loving hands that massage or help heal in some other way are always a precious blessing and must always be appreciated and celebrated, but I cannot express enough the powerful and wise uniqueness of the individual.

My thanks to the organizers for extending an invitation to travel with Healing Touch Partnerships on the '97 tour to carry the Maori teaching throughout the USA and Canada. Everything from my first communication with you has been an absolute delight, a real bonus. I thank you and honor you all. I pay tribute to you, your ancestors, all those who have passed on beyond the veil. May they be at peace. May we who continue to live on this plane, also be united in peace. As is customary in my country, I will sing you a song of peace. The ordinary meaning of "AIO" is peace, but within the realms of its sacred context we include love, joy, and truth.

AROHANUI, lots of love to you all, from Hawaiiki Tautau, the ancient name of New Zealand when she was established as the pulse of ancient Hawaiiki, the largest continent in the world, before most of it went under water, 12,000 years ago. This Motherland included Australasia. So be it!

Rangimarie Turuki (Rose) Pere
Waikaremoana, New Zealand

Unexpected Help from Rose Pere

On many occasions Rose Pere has come to my assistance. Sometimes it is in my awareness and other times it is out of awareness. I am privileged to know and be connected to Rose Pere who is a Maori *Tohuna* (healer).

After the surgery for my breast cancer, I had called Rose on the phone to talk about arrangements for her to go on tour with us in the USA in 1997. After we finished our business she asked how I was doing. I told her about my surgery. She immediately asked what "color" I was. I didn't know what she was doing and hesitated, but when I went inside the color black came to me and I told her that. She then spoke some Maori language I did not understand. She asked again, "What color are you?" This time I reported, "Gray." She repeated going into her traditional language, asked the same question, "What color are you?" This time I said, "Green." She said that is good and hung up! After that healing I did not have any more tiredness associated with the surgery. What I experienced was beyond anything I knew to do and it taught me once again, there is no one path to healing!

Another time I was getting ready to attend a very challenging meeting at an international conference of which I was on the Board of Directors. As I was preparing to go to bed Rose appeared to me. I could see her and hear her voice say, "Oh, so you need to have your back covered!" I laughed and thought I didn't even call for her help! I told my friend about the experience that night. The next morning when I was eating breakfast with a group of friends and told them the story, as I was relating it, she appeared once again. This time she appointed two Maori men in traditional dress with spears to stand on either side of me. She placed herself behind to protect my back! Needless to say, no one messed with me at that meeting! Seriously, all went well and I felt very protected.

What I learned is that once you connect energetically with a healer, there are times they come to visit you in times of need, out of awareness. Several people have reported this phenomena to me over the years that I come to visit them unexpectantly. Now I know why!

Mary Jo Bulbrook
Carrboro, North Carolina

Maori Teachings

The teachings of the Maori tradition are taken from my experiences in studying with and being with Rose Pere over the years. Below is recorded a few of those in English that I would like to report.

Peace, Love, Joy, Truth to the Universe.

Spirituality governs and influences the way we interact with others.

Respect all people.

May the violet flame, the spirit of freedom that upholds justice and truth prevail.

Children are the greatest legacy we have.

Use the gift of love if anything negative affects your life.

Unconditional love is essential to the survival and total well-being.

Language is empowering and the life line and sustenance of a culture transmitting values and beliefs.

Respect the Divine nature in a person.

Kinship network gives a feeling of belonging and part of value and security.

No culture is better or worse then another.

A child follows an ancient path that guides his/her life.

Emotions serve all life.

Find means, rights, and rituals to pass on the culture.

Free the self from any quality or condition that restricts the self.

Mary Jo Bulbrook
Carrboro, North Carolina

THE CALL TO SOUTH AFRICA

Meeting Credo Mutwa, Renowned Zulu Healer

After a tedious long ride to South Africa from the U.S. I was met at the airport and taken immediately to the home of Credo Mutwa. I had no idea who he was and the importance of what was about to happen to me. While making plans for this trip I had put out there that I wanted to meet some native healers of South Africa. Little did I realize that it would all come true so suddenly!

I was guided into the home of Credo and taken into a room where Credo was waiting for me. I was so unprepared for this experience, as I did not know it would happen and I had definitely not expected it to be after the demanding plane trip. I was so bummed out that I did not have a clue what to say. He asked me what I wanted to know. I innocently said, anything he wanted to tell me. When in doubt, punt!

Credo began to share an incredible description of his beliefs as a *Sangoma*, a native healer of his people. I was dumbfounded at the similarities in the beliefs between his holistic approach and that of mine. I don't know what I expected but I did not expect to be hearing myself through his words! I was struck by the similarity of his work and plight to get native healers accepted into traditional health care. His work connected deeply with ancient teachings that are now trying to be done in cooperation with Western medicine. It seems we are more alike than different.

Having spend over two hours talking with him, I asked him before I left what I could do for him since he was so generous in helping me. He asked me to pray for him. I eagerly agreed to do so, saying I did a meditation before my groups and would include him in that process.

As I got ready to leave I decided to comment on the many spectacular artifacts that were on the counter behind him. I said, "I bet these have a lot of stories to tell." He laughed and said they did. He proceeded to tell me about them, first naming a mask called the "earth mother mask." He then went to a stone in an iron box. He said that he only opened the case up that morning to do a meditation with the stone. As he was continuing to tell me about the stone's origin I heard a voice from the stone tell me it wanted to speak to Credo. I wondered how would I say that to Credo, as he didn't know anything about me and would think I was crazy! But I had a nagging feeling that I should do it and told him that the stone had a message for him and asked if he like me to give it to him.

He said yes, so I placed my hand on the stone and turned away feeling very awkward and self-conscious as I began to give him the message. It said things about his personal life as well as encouraging him about his life's work.

After I finished, I turned to see his reaction. He was grinning from ear to ear. He said that when he was given the stone which stood in front of a Hebrew temple at the door, he was told, "A woman from far away would come and make the stone speak!"

Spiritual Guidance for My Work in South Africa

That night I was awaken during the middle of the night at 2:30 a.m. I just attributed it to a time zone problem and hoped I would soon drop off to sleep. Suddenly I heard the words, "Oh Divine Master, may our people be healed." I thought that didn't sound like casual conversation. Perhaps I should get up and record what I was hearing! As I reread what I wrote I realized it was a beautiful prayer and I attributed it to the request from Credo to pray for him. I excitedly took it to the HT Course I was teaching in Johannesburg and read it during the morning meditation. After reading it I silently asked for a guide for my work in South Africa. Immediately Credo appeared over the group, wrapped his cloak over the group, and I knew that his Spirit would guide me. (The prayer is listed at the end of this book.)

That night I was again awakened at the same time and I saw wooden boxes all lined up besides themselves. They looked like coffins to me and just as I had that thought the lids opened and a skeleton came out. I saw Credo off to the side and he said, "Our spirits need to be healed as well."

I left with a friend to go to Skukuza to a game reserve and onto Capetown for more teaching. On my return to the U.S. I was routed through Johannesburg. I was standing in line to go through customs when all of the sudden I was filled with an intense light that came up through my entire body very rapidly. I said to myself, "What just happened to me?" Just then, I saw Credo's spirit in front of me in his traditional robes and he bowed to me. As I tried to digest what just happened to me, I heard a lot of noise behind me. I turned to see what all the commotion is all about and I saw the room filled with African Spirits all laughing and smiling, waving good-bye and asking me to come back.

Needless to say, I was dumbfounded regarding all of these experiences and know that my life will never be the same. I don't know how it will all evolve, I only know to, "just walk the path."

Mary Jo Bulbrook
Carrboro, North Carolina

Travelling with Mary Jo in South Africa

My journey to Ulusaba actually started the year before when I met the manager of Ulusaba on the Rovos Rail, "The Pride of Africa," on a trip from Pretoria to Cape Town. In conversation we were talking about healing modalities. I expressed my interest in traditional healing methods and told him about my experiences with the Aboriginal people in Australia when on tour with Mary Jo Bulbrook. He then invited me to visit Ulusaba and he would organize us to meet with the local traditional healers. A year later I faxed Ulusaba and accepted his invitation. The manager I had spoke to had left, but the new staff were very keen for us to come and visit the lodge. I heard no further about what arrangements they had made about meeting with traditional healers.

I met with Mary Jo a day after she had met with Credo Mutwa. I was very envious of this experience as he is very renowned in South Africa for bringing traditional healing to the notice of the Westerners at the risk of his own life and that of his family. Travelling with Mary Jo can be like a whirlwind and there generally is not much time to touch down. This is what happened in Johannesburg, where we shared experiences with the people who came to our workshops. We then flew onto Ulusaba where the driver who met us at Skukuza Airport to transfer us to the lodge kept us in suspense. He revealed as we travelled to Ulusaba that he had searched far and wide to find a bona fide sangoma for us to meet and that they were waiting for us at the lodge. I was very touched and very excited as this is an unusual event as well as an unusual request for visitors to the lodge who usually go there to see the wildlife. On our way through the Kruger National Park we saw animals which you would normally only spot after a many hours of touring around and felt that this was very auspicious for our visit. Our first sighting at the lodge was the elephant, which is known in folklore as wisdom.

Our driver was our interpreter. We then had to negotiate with the sangoma and his three assistants what would take place for the time we were to be at the lodge and to clear up the confusion about our purpose. They thought we wanted to consult the sangoma for health purposes. We were able to establish that we wanted to exchange healing experiences and methods. From that point on it was game viewing early morning, bush medicine training with the sangoma and his assistants mid-morning, a shared lunch, and a then Healing Touch demonstration in the afternoon with all the lodge staff as well as the sangoma and his assistants. We then were given the African version of a tarot card reading with the sangoma throwing the bones for a few volunteers. This created great hilarity among the staff. We had to make do with the interpreter translating our own reading and also telling the sangoma what we were doing. As we all know, energy has a universal language. The joy and amazement which ensued was a delight to see. I was personally amazed how easily the African folk took to Healing Touch, giving support to my theory that African and Aboriginal people think more with the right side of their brain than the left.

During our stay we became aware of the great misfortunes Ulusaba had to suffer in the past few years. The most recent was a lightning strike to Rock Lodge which burned it to the ground, and then a bush fire which occurred just before our arrival.

Our local guide, who we discovered had been sought as a child to do the training as a sangoma but chose to put it aside for the interim, asked Mary Jo and myself if we could be of any help to heal the land. So early next morning before flying out, we were taken to Rock Lodge, which has a stunning view over the escarpment, to feel the land and communicate with the troubled land. Mary Jo was able to communicate with a woman who proceeded to tell us that the land and the ancestors needed to be honored. We then discovered that several of the ancestors were buried below us on Game reserve land, which excluded the local people from accessing their ancestor's gravesites. Once the ranger knew what had to be done, he felt more comfortable about his mission. He told us that they used to hold a special ceremony on the rock we were standing on and that he would encourage his people to resume the ceremony to appease his ancestors and hopefully heal the land.

Jenna Vos
Byron Bay, Australia

Spiritual Teachings from South Africa

My time in South Africa was profound before, during, and after! I never cease to be amazed at the call of the Spirit to such far away places. I am humbled how a native mid-westerner would be called to service in such unusual ways. Following is a list of a few of the teachings I want to pass on to you from my time in South Africa.

Healers are often chosen by the ancestors and called to service. Many times this calling is dormant for a number of years and only becomes evident as one starts the work or has becomes very ill and Western medicine does not help.

The land, animals, and the people live in harmony. What affects one affects the other.

Rituals and ceremony are important in the healing traditions.

Ancient traditions are rich and provide support for today's Western medicine.

The land provides medicine for healing.

Love and forgiveness are essential ingredients to health.

Animals watch over the people and guide them.

African ritual and tradition are passed down through the elders.

Paying respect and homage to the elders is expected.

Survival is related to connection of all things living in harmony and balance.

Ancient wisdom is available for those who commit to serve the Higher Wisdom.

Healers function under the highest of calling and operate under a Code of Conduct.

Prayer is an important resource to add to one's life.

Mary Jo Bulbrook
Carrboro, North Carolina

A HEALING PRESENCE AROUND THE WORLD

Sharing Our Light: Healing Tours, 1994-99

Healing Touch Partnerships, Inc. is celebrating its sixth year of offering tours related to healing the self, others, and the land. Over time many magical things have happened that have influenced lives on multiple dimensions. My goal is to highlight some of them to give you a taste of the experiences of our traveling spiritual community of healers.

In 1993, Donna Duff and I brought Healing Touch to Australia, having borrowed money to do so because we believed in the work. We offered our first course in Perth, Western Australia, a HT Level I weekend in July, and then HT Level IIA the following weekend. I realized at that time if we were to develop a country we needed to find a better way of doing it as it would take forever at this rate. I returned in February 1994 and taught the next levels and repeated the Level I. Since I had so much fun, met Bob Randall and was invited to teach his people, I believed it was time to bring others to share in the wonderful experiences I was having. Thus, the idea of "tours" was born. I started telling my travel stories and inviting people to join me. We soon had our first tour group of 9 people traveling in Fall 1994.

Parallel to this planning, I helped to form the Holistic Nurses' Association of Australia in Perth, Western Australia, while I was a visiting Professor in Nursing there in 1991. After the initial forming of the Association in December 1991, they continued to meet and grow. They later sponsored me to come to Australia to offer HT. I encouraged them to go national with the organization, which they did. I had the privilege of being the keynote at that first conference and brought the "traveling spiritual community" with me. Although we would not have used that term then, the description emerged as I evaluated what happened as we gathered together and shared our light wherever we went. We combined networking healers with offering the HT curriculum, and provided a viable framework to prepare HT practitioners in Australia and New Zealand.

I realized in the planning stages of the first tour that I needed to create an organization to handle my work which had evolved beyond merely teaching the HT courses. I was now involved with working with native people in their own country, helping to network healers, and assisting in the healing of the land as well as spirits of the land.

I had cared for a monk for several years. During that time I visited him at his monastery in Western Australia. I had visions of healing work that needed to be done there and was guided to bring a group of healers to the monastery. Mary had visited me about helping with healing. As I made a visit to the monastery, I commented on a statue of Mary that was displayed in a cabinet in the front entrance of the meeting place. It turned out that the monk I worked on had been given that statue when he was ordained a new priest. Since priests do not own anything, he had given it to the monastery. It was placed in the entrance for others to share in its beauty. The importance and significance of connecting with Mary in this way struck me as I felt she was calling us to do healing there. Little did I realize what that meant until the tour group came in the Fall of 1994.

The group went to the monastery and we were guided to go to the orphanage that was run by the monks for the Aborigine children who had been taken away from their parents. There were trapped spirits of the mothers of the children found wailing in despair at the inability to be with their children. The government had wronged the Aborigine people and family life was destroyed by the disruption of the family unit that was so important to the Aborigines. This event became very significant to me as it was the first time I had participated in healing of spirits on a large scale. We walked through the orphanage and cleared the energies from the children as well as the mothers found at the entrance to the closed doors. The experience forever shaped my concept of religion and the need of souls on different planes of life.

In NZ we had similar experiences, but they were connected to the Maori people. We held the HT training after being invited by one of the natives to teach at her family's Maori Healing Touch. The significance went way beyond the mere event of teaching HT, as that was minor to the spiritual experiences we were having. Maori elders visited us and showed the events that had happened many years ago. My bringing the tour group of healers and students to this particular Marae removed the pain and guilt from centuries past regarding white people.

The following year, seven tour participants returned as the tour group grew to 35. This time we went to Central Australia and added the contact with the Aborigines visiting their sacred sites and establishing the energy lines of our relationship. Very quickly we became family. Our community was totally accepted by the Aborigines. We had successfully bridged the gap of generations, cultures, and color. Stories about those times would fill a volume of its own.

The third tour had a group of 25 who followed the same ritual of HT classes, networking internationally, connecting with native people, healing themselves, and fully experiencing the culture firsthand as guests of the natives.

By 1995 we were able to offer the first HT instructor's course outside of North America. Janet Mentgen and I were the first teachers of that diverse and interesting class. It was a very rich blending of energies and offered us many wonderful experiences together, including another trip to Central Australia, being taught by native healers, and visiting the HT Partnerships Property site.

We were invited to submit a paper for the International Congress of Nurses in Vancouver, Canada and that served as a focus to bring our sister and brother healers to America. So in 1997 we returned the hospitality and brought 9 Kiwi's and 15 Australians to USA and Canada. As a traveling spiritual community from May 24-July 2, 1997, our activities were a tremendous success. We brought our Partnerships in Ancient Wisdom to receptive HT communities in America.

Our journeys took us to Atlanta, Georgia; Tennessee; Cincinnati, Ohio; Scranton, PA; Virginia Beach, Virginia; Richmond, VA; Denver, CO; Olympia, WA; and Vancouver, British Columbia. Hundreds of people shared in the energies of this rich collection of healers. We did healing of the land, of the people, and of the animals. We sang together, cried together, laughed, and shared our pain and joy. It was one of the most meaningful experiences of my life.

At times there were 36 people traveling on the tour as the Americans joined us. We presented at the esteemed International Society for the Study of Subtle Energy and Energy Medicine (ISSSEEM), the American Holistic Nurses' Association, and the prestigious Congress of Nursing's 21st Quadrennial Conference in June. I organized a panel of representatives to present at this conference, which hosted 5,000 nurses from all over the world to focus on nurses, nursing, and health. It placed energy work in its rightful place, in the center of mainstream nursing.

We continued the tour tradition and in 1998 returned with a small group to our beloved Aborigine and Maori family. In January, 2000 the down under folks will join our tour group in Hawaii for the annual Healing Touch Partnerships conference. Aborigine Bob Randall and Hawaiian healers will join together for a gathering in Honolulu as well as Kauai. We will gather under the theme, "Our Hands and Hearts Connecting." Through hands and hearts connecting, we have become one unit in the light—all committed to serving and sharing our love to bring peace and harmony in the world.

Mary Jo Bulbrook
Carrboro, North Carolina

Traveler's Tales: 1996 Australia Tour

I have lived in Australia now for thirty years. Don, my husband, was born here. Neither of us had ever been to Uluru, the sacred site of the Aborigines (Ayers Rock). This trip came about because I saw the advertisement for the Healing Touch Tour to the Outback when I attended the New Zealand Holistic Nurses' Conference. Even though I have not been a student of Healing Touch, I was advised that we would be welcome to join the tour. For me, it was a *journey of the heart to the heart*. I needed to say my thanks to this land, which has nourished my children and me for thirty years.

We arrived in Alice Springs in the middle of a 44 (C) degree-day, and were greeted by Aborigine Bob Randall and some of his numerous family. He was a most gracious host and turned out to be a wonderful guide for the tour. He works for the Institute for Aboriginal Development in Alice Springs and is a great teacher of unconditional love and Aboriginal tjukurpa. He teaches by stories, songs, and example. (*Tjukurpa* is an Aboriginal word, which we interpret as Dreamtime. To Aborigines, the tjukurpa means existence in the past, present and future. From *Desert Dreaming* by Deidre Stokes.)

That last hour flying high above the endless desert has left me moved in a strange sort of way. The imprints of the red sand in all its myriad patterns, the under earth patterns of the dry river systems, were so beautiful, and so vast, they took my breath away. Now I could see the desert art from the air. It looked like the lovely dot paintings typical of the Aboriginal desert artists. They are simply painting the land they know and love so well.

Flying to Alice
  I am moved
By the vast undulating desert
    Beneath our wings
    I am moved
By the patterns of endless waves
    In the desert sea
    Stretching to infinity

  I am moved
By the curls and swirls
    And intricate lacery
    Of dry river beds

  I am moved
By the loving smiling, welcome
Of the People of this land on our arrival
And their gentle hospitality to us fringe dwellers
    From a far away shore

  I am moved

Alice Springs seems to be about 1200 kms from most other main cities on the fringes of Australia. An extraordinary oasis in the midst of this huge continent of the desert and semi arid zones. Flanked by the beautiful rugged MacDonnell Ranges, "old as the hills" took on new meaning when we were told that these hills had been higher than the Himalayas eons of time back. For the Luritja people, they are the Dreaming tracks of the great Caterpillars.

Because this tour was organized by Healing Touch Partnerships, there was an exchange of healing ways on the first afternoon. We were privileged to meet a number of Aboriginal healers and a Ngangkari, Bush Doctor, who travelled all over the Northern Territory and Central Australia. It was very special to be instructed in the uses of some of their healing plants, oils and ways and to be able to share with people of such a long lineage of healing and natural understanding of life and the land.

Their wisdom and teaching is handed on to the children by the grandparents, not the parents. In their scheme of understanding, the physical world, Human world (relationships), and the Sacred world all match and matter equally. There is no separation in their perception as there is in ours. They have the epitome of a holistic view of life and I believe we will have to be humble enough to learn it from them very soon if we are to survive the ravages of our civilization.

Bob and his family, including our coach driver, John Spencer, told us stories of the land as we passed through different areas. As they are both the products of Aboriginal heritage, as well as European, we had history from both sides of the equation. John had been a stockman and knew the plants and animals intimately. Bob had been brought up with his mother and people on the land between Tempe and Angus Downs Stations in Central Australia up to a mission station in Arnhem land. Until that catastrophic shift, he had never known what is was to have a roof over his head. The stars were his ceiling. Coming into white man's world and houses would have been a severe sensory deprivation. Both men gave us the greatest insights into the land they love. My impression is that the land heals us when we take time to listen and dwell on it, inwardly and outwardly.

Landspeak
What does the land say to the people?
Learn to listen
listen
listen
People who do not listen
Do not last
That is all.
I will still be here in 1000 years
Will you?

The lack of water is potent in its implications. Alice has good water from the deep artesian basin beneath the sands. But how long it will last at the rate it is being used is anyone's guess. They have had no decent rainfall there for two years now and some of the well-known water holes are drying out.

On the way to Uluru, we visited Rainbow Valley, the rainmaker's place—not a drop of water, not a cloud in the hot air. Next, we cut across country on a dirt road to King's Canyon. On the way, John stopped the bus for a stretch and we wandered across the hot red earth to a big desert oak. Spreading its massive branches out across the sand. As we stood there in the shade, Bob said quietly, "This is my nursery." He had lived in this part of the country with his mother. She walked the 100 miles between Tempe and Angus Downs and lived by the land in between working for the stations.

At last, we reached The Rock. Our first view of great Uluru was from the western side at sunset. Gradually the colours change as the great Being cooled down and the purple shades of light changed to deep blue night. The sand was so rich and red/brown, and so soft it felt like silk to touch. To those who don't know this land, it is often described as harsh, but when you get closer you realise it is the word fragile that should be used. Away in the distance, 50 kms away, was the purple pile of Kata Tjuta (The Olgas).

Last Sight of Kata Tjuta
Red earth
Purple rock
Sun rising
Bird calling
Tiny tracks across the sand
Every action
Leaves an imprint
Light breeze
Wind calling
Sighing, falling
Delicate vastness
Tuning my ear
My heart responding
Longing
Feeling
Singing
>   Oh Aiiiiii!

The next morning we rose at 5:00 a.m. to drive the 20 kms to catch the sunrise over Uluru. Then we did the 8 km walk around Uluru, stopping often at different points to listen and feel the power of this place. The Cultural Centre was the next stop. A beautifully designed serpentine building of natural materials full of Tjukurpa graciously explained and exhibited by the People of this Land.

That day was very hot and we were to learn that a Japanese tour guide had fallen to his eventual death off the Rock climb. It took three days and thirty people to get his body out. Tourists are asked and advised by the Aboriginal owners of Uluru not to climb their sacred rock, but still the tourist companies sell the climb and ignore the wishes of the people who know it best. Bob said quietly, "The People will be sad, they will be in mourning now this has happened again."

After the tour finished we hired a camper van and stayed on three days longer exploring the western and then the eastern ends of the MacDonnell ranges either side of Alice Springs. Our last night was spent at the invitation of our friend Bob who took us to his special land near Honeymoon Gap, where we watched the sunset and a full moon rising out of the east—"night rising" in Bob's vernacular.

Night Rising
We sit on the Land
 At sunset
The rocks are hot from the heat of the day
The birds are making goodnight roosting sounds
Crickets 'click' in amongst the dry grasses
Tiny bats dart overhead on silent wings
The breeze is soft and cool now
 The silence is palpable
 As if holding our breath
 Waiting for Moonrise
 Tonight is the Full Moon
The western sky is pricked
 By the Evening star
In the East we watch the skyline change
Deep purple melting into layers of pink and blue
A glow appears outlining the mountain top
The ghost gums sign in the soft moon breath

We watch and wait with eagerness
Listening to the silence of nightrise
 Syrius, the Dogstar
 Sparkles in the Southern sky
 Ah! The Moon comes now
Peeping over the brow of the hill
Second by second she rises and glows
 A golden magical orb
Taking up the night with her beauty

Janna Moll and Dawn McKern
Summarized Tour Group Stories

Healing Touch Song
(Written & Sung by Bob Randall, Healing Touch Partnerships Tour '97)

Touch me with your healing, heal me with your touch
Take me in your memory, I need to heal so much.
Heal me with your smile, make my life worthwhile,
Heal me with your healing, heal me with your love.

Heal me with your kindness, you give me through your eyes,
Heal me with your softness, like the waters flow,
Moving through my country, touching all the trees,
When the rain is falling, heal me with the breeze.

Heal me from a distance, from places far away,
Heal me each moment, each hour of every day.
Heal me with your closeness, hold me in your arms,
Touch me with your healing, heal me with your touch.

As we meet together, let us meet with love.
Gifts from all the spirits around us and above.
As we share together our many different ways.
May love be our healing, throughout every day.
May love be our healing, throughout every day.

The Healing Touch song was written and composed by our
Aborigine elder, Bob Randall, while on the 1997 Healing Touch
Partnerships Tour throughout the United States and Canada.
    There were 30 people traveling together from Australia and New
Zealand doing nine workshops throughout the Northeast. It was
during one of our rides in the van as we traveled from site to site that
Bob wrote this song. He taught it to us and we spent many wonderful
hours singing together, sharing our love and light in community, and
passing this on through our songs and stories.

Prayer for Unity
Oh, Divine Master
May our people be healed
May they walk in truth
Light and love
May their path leave footprints
For others to follow
May peace ring out
Throughout our land
May there be justice for all
As we live in unity
One with the Spirit,
One with the Lord
May we never falter, or waver
In the pursuit of justice
For all.

May our brothers and sisters
Throughout the world be
With us in this journey
There is strength in unity
There is purpose in unity
There is oneness in unity.

Our land, air, water, animals and plants
Need healing too, as we
Respect ourselves and respect others
Then we in turn will respect the land.
Air, water, animals, plants, all will
Be healed as we are mutually
Interdependent.
This is our prayer for unity,
The highest act of love, faith, hope
And justice for all.

Inspired by Credo Vusamazulu Mutwa,
Revered Zulu Spiritual Leader
Johannesburg, South Africa (5/17/98)

Channelled and Recorded by Mary Jo Bulbrook

EPILOGUE

On this Thanksgiving Day, 1999 I have reflected on all that has transpired this year—where I have been, where I am going, and where my work is going. The intensity of the Light behind this effort to produce *Healing Stories* has been the highlight of the year and of my career. It is the culmination of my life's work. I never intended for this book to look like it does. It was shaped by Mother Mary, through twists and turns of events all interwoven together out of consciousness connected with guidance. Dan and I followed the ebb and flow where the Light was shining. This is the first of what I hope to be many editions of sharing our stories and telling what is in our hearts. Healing of the self and others is what this is all about. We are not trying to convince anyone of anything. We are simply telling our stories!

This book seems to represent a chronology of my life and work, which are based on a call to service. We are finding a profound truth in this process of sharing our stories to each other—truth about our work, our needs, and ourselves. As we connect with our truth, things seem to fall in place, for there is unity between, among and within. The Light that shines for all to see will activate what is needed to maintain and regain health. The profound truth—as we give, we receive and as we receive, we give—has been the underlying focus and philosophy of my work. Abundance flows freely as we attune to God. With His support, Mary's, the Angels and other Spiritual beings that are there to serve and guide, there is nothing we can't do.

The future of energy work is very promising. There is no right or wrong way to progress. Everyone begins where they are and pro-ceeds from there in developing as a healer. We need never forget focusing with a beginner's mind or seeing from a child's perspec-tive. We are being guided to a new level of attunement to the Divine. We are being asked to move beyond our fears and fully connect to the Light and share what is in our hearts.

I remember the closing words from Mary from the first message she gave me in 1993. The day I received that message seven years ago falls on the same day that *Healing Stories* is due from the publisher (January 8, 2000). I believe it is also significant that the publication of this book occurs right after Epiphany (January 6th).

This day celebrates the three kings coming to see Mary and her child. The kings followed the Light and travelled from distant lands. They spoke different languages and held different beliefs, yet they were all drawn to the Light of the Divine. Mary gathers people from different cultures to honor God. I know this book is guided by Mary and I have tried to honor her guidance and energy every step of the way. I leave you with her words from that first message I received seven years ago:

Share God's truth by your beingness. Take each moment of the day to be your prayer, your offering to make this world a better place, for in doing so the "whole" will be changed. Peace starts at home—in your heart, in your being—with those you love and those who are hard to love. Once this truth is realized, this age will be transformed into a new golden age with less pain and suffering.

Service is the tool to salvation of the self and the world. Align your will, life, and love with God's. That is all you need. Pray to me and the other saints for guidance on the path. We readily await your attunement to our energies, as we are eager to instruct.

Lovingly, Mary

Mary Jo Bulbrook
Thanksgiving Day, November 25, 1999

APPENDIX

List of Contributors

Energetic Healing: Background and Code of Ethics

Healing Touch: Background

Bibliography

Glossary of Terms for Healing Touch and Energetic Healing

Healing Touch Partnerships

LIST OF CONTRIBUTORS

Abilay, Kia (San Francisco, California)
Kia is a CHTP and CNA who lives North of San Francisco. She has incorporated HT and EH with her clients and has a creekside treatment room. She is also the creator of a chakra teddy bear and coloring book.

Ashton, Sue (Pappinbarra, New South Wales, Australia)
Sue is a Registered Nurse having trained in England in the early 1970's. She currently works part-time in Community Nursing and uses Aura-Soma, Reiki, and Healing Touch in combination in her private practice. She teaches all levels of Aura-Soma training and travels extensively promoting the use of color and light for healing.

Bartlett, Charles (Surfers Paradise, Queensland, Australia)
Charles is the artist for the Southern Landscape Cross that is on the front of the *Healing Stories* book. He has worked with the Aborigines for many years and channels an Aborigine spirit. His gifted drawings come from his deep Spiritual connections with the land and the people of Australia.

Bigley, Mark (Arlington, Texas)
The Reverend Mark Bigley, M.Div., M.A., is an Episcopal Priest and uses Healing Touch in his ministry in the hospital, counseling, and spiritual direction.

Boyd, Anne (Augusta, Georgia)
Rev. Anne Boyd, CHTP/I, DIF has been a Certified HT Instructor for over six years with an active private practice in Augusta, GA. She also is a Reiki Master and conducts shaman journey workshops in Australia and New Zealand, and has interacted with native healers in both countries. She has taught HT in Romania as well. Anne has been a leader of spiritual study groups for over twenty-five years. Her angel pin designs come through Divine inspiration and are available through her business, Angelight.

Boyd, Helen (Glen Allen, Virginia)
Helen has a home based HT practice and uses her gifts with her family and friends. She completed HT Level IIIA in August, 1999.

Brown, Deny (Richmond, Virginia)
Deny is a Certified HT Practitioner and Instructor, a Registered Nurse, and a Woman's Health Nurse Practitioner. She has run a HT private practice, Energy Works, in Richmond, VA since 1995 offering surgery support, stress and pain management consultations, instructions for families, personal growth work, and more. She teaches EH Level I, Introductory HT courses, has given many professional conference presentations. Deny is available as a consultant to other practitioners who want to develop a practice or HT in their area.

Bulbrook, Mary Jo (Carrboro, North Carolina)
Mary Jo is a Registered Nurse and Certified HT Practitioner and Instructor. She is the Founder and Director of Healing Touch Partnerships, Inc., an international organization dedicated to Connecting through the Light. She developed the Energetic Healing Program (EH), and teaches EH and HT extensively throughout the U.S. and abroad. She is President of the International Alliance for Health and Healing, a non-profit organization dedicated to providing education, research, service, and leadership in health and healing. Mary Jo has a 20 year distinguished career in university teaching, administration, practice, and research in the USA, Canada, and Australia. Through her leadership Healing Touch was introduced and developed in Australia, New Zealand, and South Africa. She is on the Board of Directors of Healing Touch International and a member of Sigma Theta Tau, the International Nursing Honor Society. In 1989 she was named Canadian Holistic Nurse of the Year. She organized a symposium and presented HT Worldwide at the 21st Quadrennial Congress of Nurses in Vancouver, Canada, in June 1997. Her partnership work with the Aborigines of Australia and Maori of New Zealand has opened their ancient wisdom and teachings worldwide in the HT and EH communities.

Bulbrook, Bill (Carrboro, North Carolina)
Bill is a graduate of North Carolina State University in business management and is the business manager for HT Partnerships. He is also the Executive Director of the International Alliance for Health and Healing, a non-profit organization dedicated to providing education, research, service, and leadership in health and healing. He has taken HT Level I. It changed the course of his life.

Bulbrook, Jim (Carrboro, North Carolina)
Jim is a senior at University of North Carolina in Chapel Hill where he is majoring in math with an emphasis in physical education. He spent time traveling in Europe, Australia, and New Zealand and was part of the HT Partnerships Tours for three years. He combines his love of the outdoors with problems of science and working with people, especially children.

Cavanaugh, Sister Barbara (San Francisco, California)
Barbara Cavanaugh is a Sister of Mercy who lives and works in the inner city of San Francisco. She is an RN, CHTP, and practices Energetic Healing in the San Francisco Women's Jail and in a rehabilitation program called Standing Against Global Exploitation. Barbara spent thirty-one years in Puno, Peru, in the Andes at 12,000 feet elevation, working as a missionary, nurse and midwife. She lived simply among the native Aymara and spoke their language. She also worked with native healers and appreciated their holistic view of life.

Chvala, Mandy (Midlothian, Virginia)
Mandy is a second grade teacher from Midlothian, Virginia. She has been newly introduced to the work of energy-based health and healing and has taken HT Level I.

Clarke, Bernie (Olympia, Washington)
Bernie is a RN, MS, CHTP/I, FAAN, and the International Coordinator for the Energetic Healing Program. She practices and teaches Energetic Healing and Healing Touch. Prior to her retirement as a university professor she taught Maternal Child Nursing for over 40 years and is a Certified Pediatric Nurse Practitioner. In addition to teaching formal courses, she offers introductory workshops in healing practices in hospitals and community and church groups.

Duennes, Mary (Cincinnati, Ohio)
Mary Duennes is a Registered Nurse, and also holds Master of Arts degree with more than 25 years of experience in a variety of staff and management roles. She is a CHTP with extensive experience acute care hospital setting as well as in private practice. Mary integrates Energetic Healing with Healing Touch in her work with clients. She is a Certified HT and EH instructor and a certified Enneagram instructor. She is currently working as a Parish Nurse in Cincinnati, Ohio.

Duff, Donna (Carrboro, North Carolina)
Donna is a nurse healer, Certified Healing Touch Practitioner and Instructor, massage therapist and neuromuscular therapist in private practice at the NCCHT. She has taught HT throughout the USA, Canada, Australia, and New Zealand and is one of the faculty assisting in the training of instructors in Healing Touch. Her specialty includes pain management and combining energy work with massage therapy. Donna has a special relationship in working with seniors. Since 1987 she has offered services at Carolina Meadows, a retirement community in Chapel Hill, NC, including exercise, wellness support, grief counseling, massage, energy work, and companionship. Seniors are her extended family as she showers love, support, and care to them beyond just a professional relationship.

Duff, Gerard and Yolanda (St. John's Newfoundland, Canada)
Gerard is a high school teacher with a B.S. in St. John's Newfoundland specializing in math and science. He has taken HT Level I. Yolanda, his wife has a B.A. in Primary Education with a major in French.

Dupre, Joanne (South Dartmouth, Maine)
Joanne, MS, PT, CHTP/I has over 25 years of rehabilitation experience in the areas of orthopedics, neurology, early intervention, special education, and home care. Joanne has incorporated energy based work into every aspect of her physical therapy practice. Joanne is also Certified HT Practitioner/Instructor, a Reiki Master/Teacher, a Certified Clinical Aromatherapist Instructor, and a Cranio-Sacral Therapist. She has a private practice of Integrated Therapy. She teaches Reiki, Healing Touch, and Clinical Aromatherapy locally and throughout the United States.

Ellis, Mary (Springfield, Oregon)
Mary is a graduate of Columbia University/Presbyterian Medical Center (BSN, RN, CHTP). She has lived in Africa, Asia and Europe for 20 of the last 30 years. She initially learned energy work in Manila, Philippines, as "pranic healing." Since completing HT she has established her own practice first in the Seattle area and now in Springfield, Oregon. In her HT practice, she also incorporates EH and Reiki along with her interests in yoga, Qi Gong, herbs, and aromatherapy. She has a number of years of Hospice and home health experience.

Forman, Paul (Anakie, Victoria, Australia)
Paul is a father of three and is working full-time as a Certified Healing Touch Practitioner and as a Clinical Masseur. He lives in the bush in a small town called Anakie and also spends quite a deal of his time working with farm and native animals. He has successfully done healing on cows, dogs, kangaroos, and walla-bies. He and his family traveled with HTP in 1997 to the USA.

Givens-Myers, Jean Marie (Williamsburg, Virginia)
Jean Marie took HT Level IIIA in August, 1999 and is working in Williamsburg serving the community in their health journey.

Gress, Eileen (Apex, North Carolina)
Eileen is an accomplished musician who started playing horn at age 9. With many years of practice she got a job in a professional orchestra. She has a horse farm where she has horses, goats, cats, and dogs that she frequently works on using HT and EH. Her new passion through animal work is expanding her healing to humans. She not only brings joy and love to others through her music, but also with HT and EH (including long-distance healing).

Gustafson, Jean (Scotia, New York)
Jean is a Certified HT Practitioner and an Instructor in HT and EH. She currently works in an educational setting as a pediatric physical therapist. Her caseload consists primarily of children with multiple disabilities. She integrates energy-based health care into her physical therapy practice. Jean has worked with children throughout her career. She also has a limited private practice out of her home.

Hall, Jane (Melbourne, Victoria, Australia)
Jane is an RN, Midwife, BSciAdvNurs(Ed), FrCNA, FACM, HTP, TTP, using energetic-based healing as a key part of her practice. She is Director of Healing Dimensions which offers private practice and consultancy in healing and educa-tion. Jane is a teacher of Therapeutic Touch and conducts seminars and workshops centered around personal and professional growth for healers.

Harris, Barbara (Osprey, Florida)
Barbara is a Registered Nurse, Certified in Holistic Nursing, a Reiki Master/Teacher, a Massage Therapist, and a Natural Health Care Practitioner. She holds a B.A. in psychology. Her graduate studies include courses in transpersonal psychology, counseling, and mental health. Barbara is a past President of the National Association of Nurse Massage Therapists. She has taught Therapeutic Touch for the past ten years and has completed HT Level I and II. She has designed and chaired three national nursing conventions for nurse healers, NANMT, and AHNA. Barbara lives on the west coast of Florida with her husband Chip. Her personal and professional life has taken an unexpected turn in the writing of *Conversations with Mary: Modern Miracles in an Every Day Life*. Barbara considers this inspirational and spiritual book a culmination of her soul's work.

Herbst, Eileen (Brighton, Michigan)
Eileen is a Registered Nurse and the Coordinator for the HT Partnerships, Journey into the Light Labyrinth. She has studied spiritual and mystical traditions for many years and incorporated this work into her healing practice and spiritual ministry.

Hock, Jane (Houston, Texas)
Jane focuses her HT and EH practices with seniors and children. She assisted with the support groups in Houston having co-coordinated them for over ten years. She has a passion for the work and is committed to minister to those in need.

Jordan, Carol (Raleigh, North Carolina)
Carol is a Registered Nurse who completed her HT Level IIIB in August, 1999. She is dedicated to serve others with her gifts of humor and energy-based healing.

Karl, Debbie (Clinton, New York)
Debbie Karl has been a Registered Nurse for 20 years. She is a Certified HT Practitioner and a Craino-Sacral Therapist. Currently she has a private Holistic Nursing Practice in Clinton, New York where she lives with her family.

Keith, Rebekah (Creedmoor, North Carolina)
Rebekah has been studying and practicing energy-based healing since 1990 and has been certified in HT since 1995. She now complements that work with EH and finds this combination exceptionally useful to deal with physical, emotional, mental, and spiritual issues. She is involved with a research project at the VA Hospital in Durham, NC, and has helped introduce HT into a local hospice and in a grief ministry within her church.

Kelly, Colleen (St. John's Newfoundland, Canada)
Colleen is a Registered Nurse with a Master's degree in nursing from Memorial University of Newfoundland in St. John's where she lives and works.

Kelsall, Janeece (Geelong, Victoria, Australia)
Janeece Kelsall is a Certified Healing Touch Practitioner who also works with esoteric, spiritually guided, and intuitive healing. She has many years of experience in these fields. She practices from a healing centre in Geelong, Australia called, The Centre for the Study of Subtle Energy and Energy Medicine. Through the Centre, Janeece and her husband Colin, offer consultations in energetic-based healing, run training courses in Healing Touch and Dimensional Healing, and coordinate meditation and spiritual development groups. Janeece and Colin also write and edit a well-respected magazine called, *Spiritual Links* that is distributed throughout Australia. *Spiritual Links* covers a wide range of subjects on the environment, health, healing, and spirituality. It is known as the, "thinking man's guide to spirituality." Janeece and Colin are also the Australian partners for Healing Touch Partnerships in Australia.

Kemp, Jeff (Sebastopol, California)
Jeff lives and practices EH and HT in the San Francisco Bay area.

Klinger, Mary (San Francisco, California)
Mary is a massage therapist who incorporates energy work in her practice.

Klumpers, Marijke (Hawkes Bay, New Zealand)
Marijke is currently the Healing Touch Partnerships New Zealand Partner. She has an active practice combining Spiritual Healing, HT, Toning and Massage. Spirit taught her healing many years ago before coming in contact with Healing Touch. She now uses both in her Healing Practice, which she calls, "Release and Attunement to the Divine, a Process of Spiritual Remembering."

Kinney, Carol (San Anselmo, CA)
Carol is a Certified Holistic Nurse, Healing Touch Practitioner/Instructor and Massage Therapist as well as a Reiki practitioner. Her nursing career spans 38 years. She has an extensive background in psychiatry, home and hospice health care, Healing Touch, and Energetic Healing. Carol has coordinated classes for Healing Touch since 1990 and began her private practice in 1991. She sees clients throughout the Bay Area as well as lectures and teaches locally and nationally. She co-created the Mill Valley Healing Touch Clinic, four years ago, which provides healing, training for Energetic Healing Practitioners and a community service in Healing Touch and Energetic Healing.

Komitor, Carol (Highlands Ranch, Colorado)
Carol is a Certified Massage Therapist, a Certified HT Practitioner/Instructor, and a Certified Hospital Based Massage Therapist. She is the Founder and Director of the Healing Touch for Animals/Komitor Method of Healing Program (HTA/ KMH). Carol has been teaching HT nationally since 1991. She is on staff at the Colorado School of Healing Arts in Lakewood, CO, where she teaches massage students how to integrate HT with massage therapy. In 1996, Carol combined her HT knowledge and practice with a 13-year background in the veterinary profession to launch the HTA/KMH Program which is being taught across the U.S. and Canada. She also currently runs an active HT, distant healing, and massage practice in the Denver area. Carol considers herself blessed for being able to share her work through teaching and a practice that includes humans and animals.

Kubel, Katherine (Chapel Hill, North Carolina)
Katherine Kubel created the cover for the book and is the designer for many of the publications for Healing Touch Partnerships. Her business is called Print To Fit.

Lallier, Joan (Burlington, NC)
Joan is a hospice nurse who has worked for many years with patients making their transition. She completed IIIB in August, 1999 and continues to serve the dying with sensitivity, care, compassion and love.

Larrimore, Deborah (Winston-Salem, North Carolina)
Deborah Larrimore, RN, LMT, CHTP is currently in private practice as a Holistic Nurse providing the Healing Art of Touch. She utilizes Healing Touch, therapeutic massage, reflexology and acupressure as modalities of healing. Deborah's traditional nursing role includes 15 years of critical care experience in ICU, and four years as Nurse Educator for Hospice. She currently resides in Winston-Salem, NC offering an integrative holistic practice.

Leduc, Elly (Olympia, Washington)
Elly is a Registered Nurse, a Certified Healing Touch Practitioner and a Certified Infant Massage Instructor. She has had a private practice in Healing Touch since 1993 and also uses the Energetic Healing with her clients. She has experienced breast cancer herself and is facilitating a group for women who are interested in exploring growth through their challenge with breast cancer. In 1996 she produced the beautiful and inspirational instructional video, "Baby Massage, a Video for Loving Parents."

Letke, Kathleen (Chapel Hill, North Carolina)
Kathleen is a Psychiatric Clinical Nurse Specialist who has a part-time private practice integrating psychotherapy, Healing Touch, and Energetic Healing. She also uses energy work in her practice as a home health psychiatric nurse.

Mack, Cathy (Garner, North Carolina)
Cathy is a Registered Nurse, a Certified as Holistic Nurse through the American Holistic Nurses' Association, and a Certified HT Practitioner and Instructor. She maintains a private practice in Garner, NC utilizing the concepts of Holistic Nursing, Healing Touch, and Energetic Healing. Her specialty is working with seniors at the Garner Senior Center. She lectures and teaches Holistic Nursing, Healing Touch, and Energetic Healing. Since 1995 Cathy has been the coordinator of the Healing Touch classes through the North Carolina Center for Healing Touch including the study groups in Healing Touch.

Mitchell, Gerry (Atlanta, Georgia)
Gerry is as an Energy Field Therapist. With an extensive repertoire for restoring vitality by using bodywork as the primary tool, he has become a long term survivor living with AIDS and thrives in sharing that expertise in community. He combines his training as an Occupational Therapist, Health Fitness Instructor, Reiki and HT Practitioner, and Massage Therapist with herbs, nutrition, and exercise physiology in a private practice in Atlanta. He also regularly facilitates classes in The Artist's Way, kick boxing, Labyrinth meditation, sacred space, strength training, and yoga. He also facilitates a Care Team for those challenged with chronic illness and functions as a midwife to the dying.

Moll, Janna (Highlands Ranch, Michigan)
Janna is the International Development Coordinator for HT Partnerships along with being an instructor in the EH Program and a Certified HT Practitioner and Instructor. Janna is the Volunteer Coordinator for the Colorado Center for Healing Touch, coordinating practitioners to assist others in trauma within the Denver area. In addition she teaches Cutting The Ties That Bind, and has a private practice in Highlands Ranch. Janna recently moved to Colorado from Melbourne, Australia where she owns the Melbourne Centre for Healing Touch. While living in Australia for over two years she traveled with HTP studying indigenous healing with the Aborigines and Maori of Australia and New Zealand. Janna also works with the Healing Touch for Animals program.

Parker, Annis (Christchurch, New Zealand)
Annis Parker, ADN, Ed.D., is a New Zealand Registered Nurse, and a Certified HT Practitioner and Instructor. Her practice involves people from all age groups and conditions both within and outside the hospital setting. She also works with animals, especially horses, cats, and dogs. Since Annis lives in the South Island of New Zealand and is the only instructor there, she often travels to teach and work with people and animals. Her clinic practice is now run out of a separate venue, which includes counselors, massage therapists and an orthobionomy practitioner. Annis is also the Director of the Natural Health for Animals Program offered through HTP.

Pattinson, Susan (Beechwood, New South Wales, Australia)
Susan is an Interior Designer, Masseur, and HT Practitioner. She consults for Arcoessence Architects, and is one of the owners of a natural therapy centre in Wauchope known as "Essential Being." She is also married with three children.

Pattinson, Craig (Beechwood, New South Wales, Australia)
Craig is an Architect, and part owner of a natural therapy centre in Australia known as "Essential Being." His passion and goal is to create buildings which support the well-being of people. He sees the interconnectedness of all things and believes buildings and the surrounding landscape can powerfully effect who we are. His form of architecture has become known as "Arcoessence," which means getting to the core or essence of the needs of both a client and the landscape.

Pere, Rangimarie "Rose" (Waikaremoana, New Zealand)
Dr. Rangimarie (Rose) Pere, CBE, CM, is an International Educationist and consultant through Universal Rose Enterprises. She is a Maori Tohuna and has taken her work to USA, Canada as well as throughout Europe and linked into Kosova. In conducting workshops and sharing ancient teachings throughout the world she is fulfilling her mission as Elder and Tohuna in order to heal the land, people, and animals including lost or grounded souls. She believes that every person and every culture is sacred. Rose is holder of the 1990 New Zealand Commemorative Medal and was honored in 1996 as a Commander of the Most Excellent Order of the British Empire. She also attained a Doctorate of Literature at Victoria University of Wellington, NZ in 1996. She sends AROHANUI, lots of love to all, from Hawaiiki Tautau, the ancient name of NZ.

Protzman, Lori (Aiea, Hawaii)
Lori is a RN, BSHCA, CHTP. She is the Perinatal Nurse Manager for Kaiser Permanente, Hawaii and started the HT volunteer program at the medical center in 1997 with money from a grant to develop the program and conduct research at the facility. Research is underway studying HT with breast cancer patients. She is also on the advisory council for Bosom Buddies Hawaii, a service program matching HT practitioners with breast cancer patients recently funded by HTI and other local health care agencies

Randall, Bob (Alice Springs, Central Australia, Australia)
Bob Randall is an Aboriginal elder of the Pitjantjatjara nation of Central Australia, and one of the registered owners of Uluru, one of Australia's most sacred sites. He was taken from his family at an early age by the government and never saw his mother again. He grew up in Arnhem Land where he was introduced to traditional Aboriginal culture by the Iwaidja, Gumatj, and Kunwinku nations. Bob is a master storyteller, songwriter, healer, and keeper of the ancient wisdom. In 1999 he was named the Indigenous Person of the Year. He is family to Healing Touch Partnerships and has kin all over the world as we all connect together as one.

Robertson, Margaret Clare (Gisborne, New Zealand)
Margaret has practiced natural healing for 16 years after having been introduced to complementary therapies through a head-on collision in 1981 that left her with physical limitations the physicians said would not heal. Her search for care led her to energy work and HT. She runs a clinic at her home and is a member of the NZ Charter of Healing Practitioners and on the NZ Drugless Therapists Register. Margaret accompanied HT Partnerships tour to the USA.

Rulf, Barbara (Springfield, Virginia)
Barbara is a Healing Touch Practitioner with 25 years as a student and practitioner of esoteric studies and energy work. She currently has a home-based practice in northern Virginia, Healing Touch of Springfield, Virginia. Barbara's interest is in the integration of healing work with individuals and groups, most particularly through a community clinic.

Sinnett, Kathy (Detroit, Michigan)
Kathy Sinnett, RN, HNC, CHTP/I is a board member of HT International and senior faculty in the HT and EH Programs. In 1992 Kathy established a Healing Touch clinic for the supervision and practice of HT which continues to be used as a model today. She has been teaching energy medicine since 1993 at Wayne State Medical School as part of their program of Alternative Medicine. She is also head of The Michigan Center for Healing Touch, and The Sinnett Institute of Holistic Learning. She is currently developing the program to teach Spirit Release. Her full-time private practice consists of working with private clients, teaching, writing, singing, and enjoying life.

Stonack, Nancy (Tacoma, Washington)
Nancy is a Clairvoyant, CHTP, and RN who has 15 years experience in Critical Care and Hospice. Nancy is able to clairvoyantly see auras, chakras, guides, spirits, angels, past lives, congestion, and disease in the energy fields. Nancy incorporates her abilities into her private practice as a Medical Intuitive. She believes that everything is energy and therefore everything can be "read" energetically. She also firmly believes we are only limited by our personal beliefs. Her passion is challenging this belief system and encouraging others to tap into their own hidden wealth of ability and knowledge. Nancy lives in Tacoma, Washington where she uses her abilities both in her nursing and in private practice.

Stouffer, Joan (Cincinnati, Ohio)
Joan Stouffer, CHTP, M.Ed. has retired from a sensory and consumer research career at Procter & Gamble and established an active Healing Touch/Energetic Healing practice in Cincinnati, Ohio. She has focused on alleviating chronic health problems energetically as well as acute surgical pain management. Joan has also studied Cranial-Sacral, Healing Ministry, Aromatherapy, and Feldenkrais Energy disciplines to enhance holistic healing. She is a Healing Touch volunteer for TriHealth at Bethesda North Hospital and gives demonstrations and lectures for church, school, professional, and community groups.

Stouffer, Don (Cincinnati, Ohio)
Donald C. Stouffer, is a Ph.D. and CHTP. Professor Stouffer is Research Director for Energetic Healing Partnerships and the International Alliance for Health and Healing. He retired from the faculty of Engineering at the University of Cincinnati in December, 1999. He is conducting research on several methods to measure the effect of an energy treatment and the influence of scar tissue on the energy field. He has an active energy practice in Cincinnati, and is very interested in developing and understanding new treatment modalities in energy-based care.

Trollinger, Dan (Durham, North Carolina)
Dan holds an M.Div. from Yale University and is the editor of this book, *Healing Stories*. He is a freelance editor/writer, Reiki Master, and HT Practitioner with a private practice in Durham and Raleigh, NC. He also teaches "finger medicine" (what his 3 year old calls energy work) to his three young daughters, as his wife Kathleen completes her Master's degree as a Nurse Practitioner in Cardiology.

Wander, Carol (Woodinville, Washington)
Carol Wander is a RN, MBA, CHTP, and Asst. Director at a multi-hospital Regional Business Office and nurse consultant. Her healing practice consists of volunteer work at a convent, practice group (heal the healers), and working on injured dogs and birds, neighbor children, and colleagues at work.

Velting, Abby (Detroit, Michigan)
Abby is an 11 year old student at Power Middle School. She has taken HT for Animals and feels a call to work with animals in Africa.

Vos, Jenna (Byron Bay, New South Wales, Australia)
Jenna is a HT Practitioner and Instructor living in Australia, but is a native of South Africa. She has assisted with the development of HT Partnerships energy-based healing work in South Africa which involved our working with the native healers and connecting with the animals. She currently is living and working in Byron Bay while serving as a marketing agent for Rovos Rail, a Luxury Train in South Africa.

Webber-Martin, Cath (Queenscliff, Victoria, Australia)
Cath has spent many years as a student of the Ageless Wisdom. Her focus is healing, meditation, and the link with the psychology of the Soul. The influence of the Soul upon the personality is her primary area of study, teaching, and practice, which incorporates intuitive and esoteric principles. She is also a Certified Healing Touch Practitioner and Instructor, Esoteric Healer, and practices Spiritual Healing. Cath has developed and teaches Dimensional Healing, which is a course in advanced training incorporating spiritual, intuitive, and esoteric teachings.

Weinstein, Roger (Atlanta, Georgia)
Roger is a Healing Touch practitioner living in Atlanta. Along with energy work he particularly enjoys music and Russian literature. He is on the HIV/AIDS team of HT Partnerships helping to research effective ways to manage and heal the effects of this health challenge.

Wood, Gayla (Chatham, Virginia)
Gayla is a Registered Nurse with over 25 years of hospital nursing experience in Critical Care, Surgery, Drug Rehabilitation, and Oncology. Currently she works at Duke University Medical Center as an Oncology Nurse. She teaches continuing education in Oncology, Healing Touch, and Energetic Healing. She is a Certified HT Practitioner and Instructor with a private practice in Chatham, VA and Durham, NC. Gayla is also the coordinator of the HT support group in Carrboro, NC for HT Partnerships.

ENERGETIC HEALING

What is Energetic Healing?

Energetic Healing (EH) promotes Healing through the Light and grew out of Dr. Mary Jo Bulbrook's distinguished university career, research and practice as a holistic nurse. It was first presented under the name Healing From Within and Without (HFWW) in 1986 at the International Nursing Diagnosis Conference in Calgary, Alberta, Canada. In 1997 the name was changed to reflect the shift to primarily energy-based interventions. EH influences the human energy system in which the body, emotion, mind and spirit are cleared, balanced, and energized thus promoting self-healing.

What is the Energetic Healing Program?

The Energetic Healing Program consists of five advanced eight-hour classes. Continuing education units are offered through the nursing profession, however the courses are open to anyone with the desire to use the heart and hands to help another person, animal or plant in distress or disease. The Energetic Healer operates under a Code of Ethics to guide the interventions.

Part I: Clearing the Internal Self
From an in-depth analysis of the individual's energy system, interventions to facilitate body, emotion, mind, and spirit healing are explored.

Part II: Identifying & Healing Wounds
Our lives are limited by physical, emotional, mental or spiritual wounds that are stored energetically either currently or other time frames, recent past or early childhood. Learn to alter the pattern(s) to become who we were fully meant to be.

Part III: Changing Belief Systems
Beliefs are stored energetically in the energy field. They dramatically influence how we lead our lives. Learn what beliefs are limiting your life and how to change them.

Part IV: Changing Relationships Energetically
This workshop teaches one how to change relationships by changing one's energy. It is based on assessing, evaluating, and treating relationships between persons using the seven chakra system.

Part V: Reshaping Family Energy Patterns
Family dynamics shape who we are, who we have become, and who we want to be. This course explores family energy patterns and shows ways to change them.

International Coordinator
Bernie Clarke, MS, RN, CHTP/I, FAAN
2369 Chambers Lake Lane SE
Lacey, Washington 98503 (USA)
phone/fax: 1 (360) 438-5404
e-mail: baclarke@sprynet.com

North Carolina Center for Healing Touch
Cathy Mack, RN, HNC, CHTP/I
413 Waterside Drive
Carrboro, North Carolina 27510
phone/fax: 1 (919) 779-3579
e-mail: CMackht@aol.com

ENERGETIC HEALING CODE OF ETHICS

In Energetic Healing, body, emotion, mind, and spirit are cleared, balanced and energized, thus assisting the client to self heal.

The healing contact or relationship is made between the healer and healee by a co-creation of meaning. Through this relationship, the energy system is assessed of the client's needs. From this data an energetic diagnosis is made to determine the appropriate interventions to support the client's return to health. After the intervention, an evaluation is made to determine the outcome of the energetic care and appropriate follow-up.

The client's permission for care is required and he/she is given information to make informed decisions regarding energy work as part of a person's health regime. The language used to describe energetic care is appropriate to the ability of the client's need and personal situation.

The principle of "Do No Harm" guides all work.

Confidential records are kept and care is documented and kept in a safe, secure space so that the individual's identity and situation is not compromised in any way.

Individuals are not discriminated against because of race, sex, creed, religious beliefs, illness, social/cultural situations or sexual orientation. The person is honored, treated with respect, and his/her privacy is maintained.

A sacred space is created for the healing whether it take place in the client's home, healer's home or office, hospital or agency setting, or in the case of an emergency, at the scene.

This work compliments traditional care. The client is encouraged to maintain his/her regular medical care. Referrals are made as appropriate. All care is coordinated with others as appropriate, respecting the wishes of the client who is in charge of his/her care.

A fee for service may be charged that is reasonable and based on the background and training of the practitioner who practices within the scope of one's background and training. EH therapists and their career path or calling are required to meet all obligations to practice in the community and setting of choice.

Supervision is available for care given, through HTP and EH peers who assist as the need arises.

The Energetic Therapist maintains high standards in providing care and practices under this Code of Ethics. All care contributes to the ongoing development of energy-based treatments.

HEALING TOUCH

What is Healing Touch?

Healing Touch (HT) is an energy-based therapeutic approach to healing. It uses touch to influence the energy system with a goal to restore harmony and balance in the energy system. HT is a collection of energy techniques drawn from a variety of sources. HT was developed by Janet Mentgen for the American Holistic Nurses' Association from her nursing practice. Healing Touch was originally designed for nurses. However, it is now open to others who have the intent to help another in their healing. Due to the growth of HT, Healing Touch International, Inc. (HTI) was formed in 1996. HTI currently provides certification for Healing Touch Practitioners and Instructors and promotes the HTI Code of Ethics and Standards of Practice to ensure high quality care. HTI is also a membership organization for the Healing Touch community.

Dr. Bulbrook is co-author with Janet Mentgen for the two textbooks that are used for the Healing Touch Programs, a senior instructor for the Healing Touch Program, and also serves on the Board of Directors for Healing Touch International.

What is the Healing Touch Program?

The HT Program is a multi-level basic energy-based program taught by certified instructors in a curriculum of 120 hours of study (Level I, Level IIA, Level IIB) plus documentation of practice (Level IIIA, IIIB). After completion of the program, the practitioner is eligible to become a "Certified" Practitioner through Healing Touch International, Inc.

Level I : Introduction and development of practice.
Level IIA & IIB: Advanced practice.
Level IIIA & IIIB: Healing Touch Practitioner (HTP) training.
Level IV: Healing Touch Instructor training.

For more information contact:

Healing Touch International, Inc.
12477 West Cedar Drive
Lakewood, Colorado 80228 (USA)
phone: 1 (303) 989-7982
fax: 1 (303) 980-8683
e-mail: HTIheal@aol.com
www.healingtouch.net

BIBLIOGRAPHY

Andrews, Ted. *Animal-Speak: The Spiritual and Magical Powers of Creatures Great and Small.* (Minnesota: Llewellyn Publications, 1998).

Baldwin, William. *Spirit Releasement Therapy.* (WV: Headline Books, 1992).

Brennan, Barbara. *Hands of Light.* (NY: Pleiades Books, 1987).

Brennan, Barbara. *Light Emerging.* (NY: Bantam Books, 1993).

Bruyere, Rosalyn. *Wheels of Light.* (NY: Simon & Schuster, 1994).

Bulbrook, Mary Jo. *Energetic Healing Notebook.* Rev. ed. (NC: North Carolina Center for Healing Touch Publishing Division, 2000).

Campbell, Joseph. *The Way of Animal Powers.* (NY: Harper and Row, 1984).

Campbell, Susan Schuster. *Called to Heal.* (South Africa: Zebra Press, 1998).

Credo Mutwa, Vusamazulu. *Isilwane – The Animal: Tales and Fables of Africa.* (Capetown, South Africa: The Struik Publishing Group, 1967).

Credo Mutwa, Vusamazulu. *Song of the Stars: The Lore of a Zulu Shaman.* (NY: Barrytown, Ltd, 1996.)

Douglas-Klotz, Neil. *Prayers of the Cosmos: Meditations on the Aramaic Words of Jesus.* (San Francisco: Harper, 1990).

Hover-Kramer, Dorothea; Mentgen, Janet; Scandrett-Hibdon, Sharon. *Healing Touch: A Resource for Health Care Professionals.* (NY: Delmar, 1996).

Lawlor, Robert. *Voices of the First Day: Awakening in the Aboriginal Dreamtime.* (VT: Inner Traditions, 1991).

Mentgen, Janet; Bulbrook, Mary Jo. *Healing Touch Level I Notebook; Healing Touch Level II Notebook.* Rev. ed. (NC: North Carolina Center for Healing Touch, 2000).

Morgan, Marlo. *Mutant Message Down Under.* (NY: Harper Perennial, 1994).

Roads, Michael, J. *Talking with Nature: Sharing the Energies and Spirit of Trees, Plants, Birds and Earth.* (CA: Tiburon, 1987).

Harris, Barbara. *Conversations with Mary: Modern Miracles in an Everyday Life.* (FA: Heron House Publishers, 1999).

Pere, Rose. *Te Wheki: A Celebration of Infinite Wisdom.* Rev. ed. (Wairoa, HB, New Zealand: Ao Ako Global Learning, 1997).

GLOSSARY: ENERGETIC HEALING

Assessment is a process to identify the current body, emotion, mind and spiritual state of health.

Aura is the energy field that surrounds all living things. There are seven identifiable layers that make up the energy system called, etheric layer, emotional layer, mental layer, astral layer, etheric template, causal body, ketheric template.

Auric Field Healing is a process to assess and treat a health challenge or wound through the energy system.

Beliefs are stored in the energy system as a result of the life experiences that shape a person.

Chakra is a Sanskrit word that means spinning wheel. It controls the flow of energy throughout the entire body. There are seven major chakras called: 1. root (physical health), 2. sacral (emotional), 3. solar plexus (mental), 4. heart (unconditional love), 5. throat (expression of self), 6. brow (visioning), 7. crown (connection to the Divine).

Chakra Assessment is determining the health status of a chakra.

Chakra Blessing is a heart to heart sharing of unconditional love through the chakra system asking for Divine intervention to assist the person to heal

Code of Ethics guides the Energetic Healing therapist and serves the client assuring him/her of the professional way in which care is delivered.

Core Star is the Eternal Source of ones Essence (Barbara Brennan, *Light Emerging*, 1993, p. 306). The Core Star is located at the center of the body and is a brilliant light shining in many colors. It can expand infinitely, radiating out through all levels of the field and influencing health and healing.

Energetic Diagnosis is identifying the presenting difficulties in the energy system of the person or animal in order to plan an intervention.

Energetic Healing is a program developed by Dr. Mary Jo Bulbrook to promote health and healing as well as to help heal and balance, body, emotion, mind, and spirit.

Energetic Reparenting is a formalized process to correct presenting energy problems from early childhood experiences.

Energy Flow is a term to describe the movement of energy through using the hands to clear blocks and balance the energy.

Energy Field Drain is a technique to clear the field of debris and replace it with healing light.

Energy Focus is adding energy to an area that is depleted.

Family Energy Healing Vortex is a process of connecting the hands to unite the energy systems together of the persons assisting with the healing.

Grounding is facilitating the client to come back into the here and now by holding the feet, gently calling the person's name, and assisting them to be well oriented to place and time.

Grounding Vitality is sending energy throughout the inside of the body through the use of the hands.

Guides and teachers are both physical and non-physical spiritual beings that help us in the process of learning and healing.

Hara Alignment is a dimension of energy composed of three parts: the ID (individuation of the person out of the void), the Soul Seat (diffuse light reaching out in all directions), and the Tan Tien (holds the physical body in manifestation). The Hara aligns to the Divine, clears the self, connects us with our hearts desire or life plan, and is grounded in the self in order to manifest and ground to the earth.

Healing from Within and Without is a holistic nursing theory that was developed by Dr. Mary Jo Bulbrook, RN, in 1986. It is the forerunner to Energetic Healing.

Healing Heart Energy uses unconditional love to heal assisting the client with forgiving and to move on with their life.

Healing Wounds is focusing on areas that have been traumatized at some time during this and other lifetimes. The impact of the trauma is stored in the energy system.

Higher Sense Perception is receiving information from beyond the five senses.

Increase Energy Flow works on moving the energy block or stuck energy in the chakras.

Inner Core Balance works on the internal energy structure of the body and functions to clear blocks and rebuild and/or repair energy lines.

Pain Release is done to drain off excess energy causing pain through the use of the hands and then replacing it with healing energy.

Restructuring Eternal Light is a process to repair the upper levels of the energy system through an advanced healing process.

Spirit is a Higher Power that guides all living things.

GLOSSARY FOR HEALING TOUCH

Centering is being fully present, connected to the self and guidance, and open to another being.

Certification acknowledgment of the completion of a prescribed program and meeting of a set of standards for a professional association.

Chakra Connection is a technique developed by Brugh Joy, MD. It's purpose is to open and balance the body's energy through facilitating the movement of energy from chakra to chakra throughout the entire body connecting all the major energy centers to flow freely.

Chakra Spread is an energy technique designed to open the chakras and produce a deep healing.

Chelation is the clearing out of the energy system of energetic debris through force from the energetic system of the healer.

Energy System has three parts (Energy Field – aura, Energy Centers – chakras, Energy Tracts – meridians) which are interdependent and influence all life. It is electromagnetic energy in a biofield, perceptible with the hands, and for some visually.

Energy Field (Aura) is the energy body around every person. In health it is a clear, vibrant, fluid, fluffy substance with lines of force that are straight allowing for an effective exchange of energy to take place. Some people can see it clairvoyantly.

Energy Centers (Major Chakras: Root, Sacral Solar Plexus, Heart, Throat, Brow and Crown) are cone shaped vortices where energy exchanges between and among the levels of the energy field. They interface with the physical body through the endocrine glands and are the master switches of energy movement and disbursement throughout the person.

Field is a condition in space which has the potential of producing a force. Field theory states that the universe is filled with fields that create forces that interact with each other.

Healer is a person giving Healing Touch or another form of healing practice who has developed the self in such a way as to positively influence the health journey of the healee.

Healee is the person receiving Healing Touch or another form of healing practice.

Healing is the dynamic process of becoming whole.

Healing Touch is energy based therapeutic approach to healing. It uses touch to influence the energy field and energy centers, thus affecting physical, emotional, mental and spiritual health and healing.

Higher Power is the name used in Healing Touch for God, the Source, Universal Energy Field, Higher Spiritual Beings.

Laser is an energy technique using the fingers to send a penetrating focus of light.

Laying on of Hands is an ancient healing technique in which the hands are placed directly on selected areas of the body and held still.

Lymphatic Drain is a fifth level intervention that works on the etheric aspects of the lymph system.

Magnetic Unruffling is an energy technique used for cleansing and clearing the complete body of congested energy including removing emotional debris and unresolved feelings.

Meditation is raising the vibrations of ordinary consciousness in order to receive higher levels of consciousness to guide one's life, clear the energy system, become centered, open, calm and focused.

Mind Clearing is a sequenced technique to assist another person to clear the mind and reach a state of peacefulness through placing the fingertips on specific areas of the head.

Pain Drain is an energy technique used to clear congestion and pain from a site that is painful.

Pain Ridge is the outer edge of where acute pain is experienced and is found in the energy field (aura) which corresponds to the pain.

Penduling is use of a dangling object to assess the client's energy field.

Scanning is a term used to indicate viewing a body part such as the aura, chakras or the physical self and noticing any indicators of energy imbalance. You can scan with the hands as well.

Sealing a Wound is the closing of traumatized areas that have resulted from an injury, surgery, cut or leak in the energy field.

Therapeutic Touch is a method (derived from the laying on of hands) of using the hands to direct human energies to help or heal someone who is ill. It was developed by Dolores Krieger, Ph.D., professor in nursing at New York University and Dora Kunz, healer.

Ultrasound is a penetrating focus of light energy channeled through thumb and two fingers. It is used for breaking up congestion, patterns and blocks.

Universal Energy Field surrounds and interpenetrates all living and non-living things. It includes highly organized geometric points of light that pulsate, and can be sensed through higher sense perception. It has an organizing effect on matter and builds form. It is what all is contained in and made from.

Unruffling is a basic healing technique in which the hands brush over congested areas needing clearing.

HEALING TOUCH PARTNERSHIPS

Healing Touch Partnerships, Inc. (HTP) is an international organization dedicated to Connecting through the Light. From classes to tours to books, every project and program sponsored by HTP is based on the model of partnership. A number of partnerships have been formed blending the expertise of each to network internationally to heal the land and people throughout the world. HTP will work in partnership with the International Alliance for Health and Healing (IAHH), a non-profit organization, 501(c)(3), tax-exempt, to continue the work described in *Healing Stories*. IAHH was founded in 1988 and is dedicated to providing education, research, service, and leadership in health and healing throughout the world.

Workshops
Healing Touch
Energetic Healing
Spiritual Retreats
Healing Land and Animals

Healing Touch Network
International Tours
Maori HT Partnership
Aborigine HT Partnership
Research Center

Teaching Materials & Products
Books, Audio & Video Tapes
Inspiration Cards, Pictures
T-Shirts, Tote Bags
Massage Tables
Journey into the Light–Pyramid Labyrinth
Pendulums, Angel Pins

Healing Touch Partnerships
413 Waterside Drive
Carrboro, NC 27510 (USA)
phone: 1 (919) 942-5214
fax: 1 (919) 968-0994
e-mail: maryjo@mindspring.com
www.mindspring.com/~maryjo

International Contacts

South Africa
Cindy Ross
PO Box 107
Merrivale, 3291 Kwazulu Natal
The Republic of South Africa
phone/fax: 27 33 330 2601
e-mail: cindyros@mweb.co.za

Canada
Liz Duff
85A Oxen Pond Road
St. John's, Newfoundland
A1B3J6 Canada
phone/fax: 1 (709) 579-6103
e-mail: eduff@calvin.stemnet.nf.ca

New Zealand
Marijke Klumpers
PO Box 8364
Havelock North, New Zealand
phone: 64 6 877 6453
fax: 64 6 877 7184
e-mail: bart.klumpers@xtra.co.nz

Australia
Janeece & Colin Kelsall
PO Box 7055
Geelong West Victoria, 3218 Australia
phone: 61 3 5223 2203
fax: 61 3 5223 2331
e-mail: Spiritual_Links@onaustralia.com.au

Call for Stories
We welcome your contributions for future editions of *Healing Stories*. Stories must relate to healing and spirituality. If you would like to share your story, please send your material to one of the addresses above. Namaste.